The School of Sacred Knowledge presents

The History of Viruses

and their Effects on Mankind and Earth

Then and Now

The Metaphysical Truths

Steven Machat

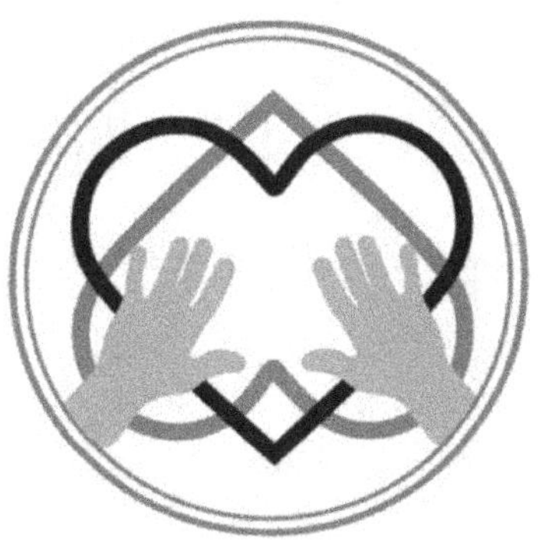

1

The School of
Sacred Knowledge

ISBN-13 : 978-1-64970-606-5
ISBN-10: 1-64970-606-5

This book is published by The School of Sacred Knowledge.
For more information about The School of Sacred Knowledge please write us
The School of Sacred Knowledge c/o Steven Machat
16673 Boca Delray Drive,
Delray Beach, FL 33484

The School of Sacred
Knowledge Series.

Metaphysical Truths.

The creation of Myths.

The Perpetuation of
those Lies.

Table of Contents

From the Author

The book you have in your hand represents all my wisdom I have gathered living on this earth as a rolling stone – A man that did not want to gather any moss.

I have lived all over our planet. I produce music and movies and have lived with the people of all cultures. Living I had to learn the truth of a medical system in each nation that I called home away from home as well as my sacred space here called today the USA.

I am a Type One Diabetic. I lived learning our bodies and the curses both from big pharmaceutical and the ancients' ways before health became a business for profits as opposed to what humans should do - this being helping each other not profiting by selling you fake foods and fake medicines saying these are the cures for all diseases.

I honor those doctors and their nurses, scientists and their students, lobbyist and the lawyers, big pharmaceutical executives and politicians as well as philosophers, poets, musicians and writers whom I have met and who helped me gain the knowledge and living wisdom I needed to be where I am today. I thank all those who married nature and understood how earth works without mankind's influence for paper profits.

I write this book now to share with you all the metaphysical truths of disease and viruses. What these are and how we can help our world and ourselves.

I show how these viruses happened in our past and what we as a mankind need to do to stop Mother Earth's revenge. I show what C19 is doing to us and how we can cure ourselves if infected and most important how to protect ourselves with the wisdom my teachers have given me on how to keep our bodies moving and staying active so we can be the men and women we wish us to be and I wish us all to be.

With time on my side during this lockdown I have studied history to find the light from our past behaviors. I share with you the message nature is sending us if we see truths. We must hear the message and correct our actions as a worldwide team and as individuals before our behavior makes the next virus that will pack a stronger punch and ends mankind.

This is Mother Earths last warning. Let's take it!

WHAT IS SCIENCE?

Science used as a noun in English we are taught, means the following: the intellectual and practical activity encompassing the systematic study of the structure and behavior of the physical and natural world through observation and experiment.

In this noun definition we are taught that science the noun, studies the physical and natural world through observation and experiment. Science in this language means the study of our physical world. Physical world means the world we see all of the animals, plants and other things existing in nature and not made or caused by people. People are not part of nature. We are led to believe nature exists to serve us, the people. We believe nature is ours for the taking.

What is the natural world in the physical noun science? Nature is the natural, physical, or material world of existence here on earth. Nature can also refer to the phenomena we experience of the physical world and also to our external physical life in general. We can then learn that although humans are part of nature, human activity is often understood as a separate category from other natural phenomena.

But please follow; Science, in reality must be taught as a verb. A verb being something that is moving and not fixed in living time. Science must be where we use the history of our knowledge to see what is happening now and how it came to change from what we assume before. If not, we will never advance until we all understand that there is always so much more to learn and share.

Science the noun is a collection of facts we are taught. A collection of past truths. We are taught these past truths are the only present answer. But they are not. Those who are taught the sacred knowledge of life understand that there is a metaphysical world. In this world you learn how life is created out of nothing at all. It is the home of how life begins. It is where we explore what's happening now and dig deep to find out why. Life is everything around us that we see and even what we do not see let alone understand. Life is magical. And all life itself begins with a virus.

In this metaphysical world of Universal and beyond realities science is a verb. The word science used as a verb becomes an active process of constant learning. The physical method of collecting data with a finite definitive conclusion is only part of the process. Things change and a true metaphysical scientist understands what they think today can be changed by a new cosmic motion of wind and water set to fire by the energy of the sun or the energy from other planets and other galaxies that collide with our planet for whatever reason. The sacred energies become additional alchemy that helps create gasses, liquids, and solids, here on Earth and even the beyond.

This book in your hands is the science of the meta-physical world and our creation of viruses. How we make new life or change our lives for all beings, not just humans here on earth.

Our World

We choke our cities with polluted skies
We could clear the air if we only try
We suck our fuel out of the earth
But we only care how much it's worth

This is our world that is dying now
This is our world to save somehow
This is our world, our world

We slay a soul for an ivory tusk
And just leave its carcass in the dust
We spear the creatures of the sea
It's a way of life so it will always be

This is our world that is dying now
This is our world to save somehow
This is our world, our world

We've changed our food's DNA
To feed more people is what they say
But the earth screams out in deathly pain
We created nothing but a viral strain

This is our world that is dying now
This is our world to save somehow
This is our world, our world

We melt the glaciers with our reckless way
We'll suffer for that and our children pay
We take what we want cause it's all about "me"
But we owe for all this cause nothing's free

This is our world that is dying now
This is our world to save somehow

This is our world, our world

If we don't care for our sacred land
And use it up with our high demand
We'll leave earth burning in an acid haze
And kill our planet with our selfish ways

This is our world that is dying now
This is our world to save somehow
This is our world, this is our world

By: Debbie Veltri

Credits

Thank you to the following:

Debbie Veltri, my editor and partner in life and light.

Brian Forbes, School of Sacred Knowledge publisher and the gentleman who told to me to write this book.

To my Yoga teachers, professors and fellow soldiers searching for truth and praying we will find justice.

To Tej Kaur Khalsa and all her devoted followers who shared their energies with me during my pre-covid 19 14 months stay in the City of the Angels.

Vladimir Megre for having the courage to write the Metaphysical series called The Ringing Cedars series which shares metaphysical truths.

To all of you be you friend or foe to never stop becoming aware.

To Socrates who I believe is my kindred spirit who had the courage to tell the Imperial Athens so called democracy that if he could not teach others to question then there is no reason to continue to live.

To our Father God, the one Creator and our Mother Earth who together gave me the gift of physical life and curiosity to examine and the strength to explore no matter what others thought about my quest.

A Poem for the Masses

Stay away, don't touch
Or else we could die
How could this happen
And do we know why

Could it be I'm sure
that this is our fault
Abusing our world
Is an all out assault

We mutate our food
And nobody cares
Cause there's no pits in our fruit
And no bugs will appear

Each cut to the ground
May bring gas and oil
But it kills us each time
We eat from the soil

What made us think
We could poison the earth
And make it all fine
If we just go to church

Stay away, don't touch
Or else we could die
How could this happen
Well now we'll know why

Debbie Veltri

Part One

Universal Naked Truths and Our Manmade Lies.

What is mankind? Mankind is human beings. Mankind is both male or female. Mankind is the human race.

Are we all equal? No. Know that truth. At birth we are endowed with DNA as well as RNA programs that makes each one of us different. How? Because in these programs of DNA and RNA we each acquire certain properties that make our individual bodies special as well as unique characters. We have many of the same characteristics, really almost all, but those differences are what controls our physical lives here on Earth.

How are we given these bodies to live in? Well we are a collection of cells that come together and live as one unit with different purposes to operate and run what becomes our personal body so our consciousness can survive and explore physical life.

How do cells come about and store the information needed so our bodies work? Well our building blocks or blue print is in our DNA which each cell must have to work.

What is DNA? DNA is short for Deoxyribonucleic Acid. This DNA is a molecule composed of two polynucleotide chains that coil around each other to form a double helix as the definition in our books of controlled learning tells us today.

This double helix, the definition goes on to say, carries the genetic instructions of the development, functioning, growth and reproduction of all known organisms and cells.

Viruses did not evolve first we are taught. We are taught viruses and bacteria are descended from an ancient cellular life form. The scientists of the noun world believe bacteria evolved to become more complex and they also believe that viruses became simpler.

We are taught today that viruses are so small and simple they can't even replicate on their own. Viruses, according to the noun scientists, carry only the essential genetic information the virus needs to be able to slip inside a host cell and coax that body's cell into making new copies of the virus as part of the hijacked DNA program and give the virus a life inside this new body. These noun scientists do not understand that a virus is a life form that can think and attack but as of yet can not really defend when the body learns and has the capability to defend and attack the virus. And we shall discover this truth as I proceed.

Ribonucleic Acid is RNA. RNA is a polymeric molecule. Polymeric means many parts. In our body it refers to the macromolecule that is composed of many parts. These parts are essential in the various biological roles in coding, decoding, regulation as well as expression of genes.

RNA has three major types of functions in our body. Function one is called mRNA. This is the messenger role. This function makes temporary copies of the information found in our individual DNA so it can be shared with the new cells, baby cells, who come to life to join our bodies.

Function two is called the rRNA or ribosomes. Here our RNA serves as the structural components of the protein making structures known as ribosomes.

The third function is tRNA. Here is how information gets transferred so the amino acids to the ribosome can be assembled to perform their life building functions.

So, what is a ribosome? A ribosome is a major key to understanding our bodies. A ribosome is a cell structure that makes protein. Protein is needed for many cell functions. Two simple examples being of the role of Proteins are they are used to a) repair your damaged cells for any and all reasons and b) direct chemical processes that your body needs to be alive.

DNA and RNA are nucleic acids. The DNA instructions make the RNA. But this as we shall learn is not how all RNA begins.

These nucleic acids with lipids, proteins and carbohydrates constitute the four major macromolecules essential for all forms of any life including viruses, I must add. A virus is a life form. And as a life form does mutate to survive. It mutates trying to find ways to stay alive in the living bodies the virus wishes to join on a permanent basis.

So, let's go and explore viruses. What is a virus?

Our dictionaries of noun scientists claim that a virus is a submicroscopic agent that reproduces only inside the living cells of the organism that houses the virus. Viruses can infect all types of life forms including microorganisms such as bacteria and archaea but not viruses. Understand this truth, a virus can not affect another virus.

So now let's learn what a virus does in metaphysical world order. A virus is probably the most abundant life form on earth. And yes, again I state that a virus is a life form. Do not listen to the noun scientists. It's ok for that to be the starting point when you learn to question conventional wisdom. Also understand most scientists called experts are really paid to say that what we know now is all there is to know ever. Different energies make new lives and end old lives. These noun scientists are really historians as they treat science as this is what is as opposed to saying this is what we now know. A true scientist is one who understands that their role in society is to discover more as change unveils a magical new truth. A new creation appears.

All life itself mutates and dissolves or evolves. We humans sure mutated from some form of earlier life to house our consciousness in this current earth-built body. I share with you how this happened and why my lifetime research on this truth is in my book Opus One The Collonization of Earth and the Making of Mankind.

The intellectual discrepancy of scientists debating if a virus is alive or is not is how a virus lives truly lives. A virus outside a cell is called a viral particle and is known as inert. Inert meaning cannot move. On its own the particle cannot reproduce itself or really do anything but look to invade a living body. And a virus will have its own life timeline to live outside a body before it dies.

A virus travels with no baggage other than the ability to hack into a cell, take over the cockpit of the molecular machinery. Once inside the victim's body the virus does live to multiply the machinery of the molecules so as to do what the virus says as opposed to the original DNA/RNA program.

And viruses have the ability to parachute out of the now infected cell body. Doing this the virus now invades other cells and creates an invasion and takes over our DNA that exists to keep us living in a program that works as planned. We become a body with a polluted wiring machine whose wires of instruction no longer work the way our DNA or RNA planned.

So, now let's go to the travel bag of a virus. I am taught by the noun scientist the virus travel bag includes a genome and a protein shell surrounding this genome.

A genome is the genetic material of an organism. It consists of DNA or RNA if the virus is an RNA virus. And I do believe that Coronavirus/Covid-19(C-19) is an RNA virus. C-19 at its birth starts as an RNA virus.

This virus comes with a cape. The cape of the virus is called a shell that helps the virus latch onto the cells of the virus's living organism hosts. Once latched the virus will climb inside that new cell's structure. The cape also helps the virus escape that cell.

Now please be aware that some of these capes are greasy. Scientists call them envelopes. These envelopes are made from the stolen shards of the previous cell's membrane.

Know this truth as history. This virus envelope is how a few virus killers of mankind's life work and do their damage to our bodies. This is the virus of new life that does affect mankind. Examples of this new life that magically appear as virus envelope killers today we call Influenza and Hepatitis C as well as Coronavirus as a group and Herpes viruses as well as HIV.

Rhino viruses which are our common cold for the most part, do not have envelopes. But saying that, the virus that causes Polio did not have envelopes either. Polio did not spread by escape. The virus was alive somewhere as is the virus of the common cold.

Envelope viruses do not like soap or water. Both soap and water do disrupt the new greasy membranes that the virus uses as its escape parachute. But once in your body you need different substances to kill the invaders.

How does a virus enter cells? It finds the hole. We are an energy force. If your energy is high that virus will have a hard time getting into your body. I will discuss this later. But if you are what I call low energy, living in fear for whatever reason, if the virus has the ability to enter your body and do damage it probably will. The virus will take up residence in the area of your body where you live the fear and have damaged parts from our life-styles including our toxins we put in earth to perpetuate something earth did not agree with in the first place.

As a sidebar, do you ever ask yourself how did my organs get damaged? If you critically analyze this question you will discover it is your life-style which you choose or which your world order creates by polluting earth with chemicals and making foods that earth did not make for our bodies to digest.

We have worldwide governments that knowingly pollute and knowingly poison us believing they can figure out a vaccine before the pollution does kill us. They knew about the birth of what we call Covid 19 and tried to have a vaccine for us as they do the flu before this pandemic hit us. Know this truth.

Our capitalistic society of corporate profits before people has damaged the parts we took from Mother Earth to live in this paradise that we have made a living hell. Climate change is caused by our polluting world industrial order. We have destroyed life that existed when our bodies were created to live and prosper on earth. We are the cancer of this planet for all living beings

I love watching us gullible conditioned fools listen to those talking climate change and giving us some wizards or witch partial remedies. We make regulations to limit our damage, but I never understood that, if you realize it is no good at all why is just a little less good. I will get to this later when I share my recommended solution. Capitalism's game is predator. The strongest survive. Nature's game is keeping everything alive as well as making sure that in the end our bodies return to earth's womb. We are the cause of Covid-19 (C19) and a lot more. This will become very apparent as I continue this story.

Now I have served the appetizer of this book, let me get to the main course of mankind's paper profit three ring circus here on earth. It's time for me to introduce the concept of Quantum Physics right now. Quantum Physics is the physics of our divided knowledge that explains how everything works. When you study Quantum Physics, you'll learn that life is a combination of matter and particles. A virus in my metaphysical awareness is none other than the smallest particle alive that is invisible to the human eye as it travels in a vibrational form looking for a host to get extended life.

Our minds could not see the virus as a solid object until we got the aid of something else. We only believe what we can see. So with the discovery of microscopes and their latest and newest inventions we can see the moving particles all around us that change our lives that we call viruses.

The viral vibrating genome is no different than our good virus by birth genome. We have an instruction kit for the production of the proteins by a good planned virus at the creation of our life in our body. A good or bad virus to survive needs to keep the proteins being made that the virus needs to survive.

The viruses can be made of DNA which is the truth for most viruses. But as I said above the virus can be made from the RNA. RNA is not as stable as DNA. It is easier to manipulate and is where most mammal infecting virus genomes are developed. The exception is herpes, I am told.

Viruses need another gene besides the canid protein which I have been calling the cape. Viruses need an enzyme known as Polymerase which the virus needs for the gene to create this substance when it tries to become the boss of your cell.

As I said previously RNA is single strand. This single strand makes RNA easier to invade as DNA is double stranded. So, Viruses attack the mRNA and distort the original birth message on this hijacking of the cells of our body temple.

I will now share with all some examples of RNA Virus for your intellectual digestion. Those viruses are the following: Hepatitis C, Influenza A. Measles, Morbillivirus, Human Orthopneumovirus.

We also have experienced RNA Viruses we call the Middle East Respiratory Syndrome as well as Rabies Virus, Dengue Virus, West Nile Virus, Vaccine Virus, Influenza B, Yellow Fever, Human coronavirus NL63 and 229E, Ebola and of course our current killer C19.

So again, I ask what does a virus do? A virus changes the host set of instructions that give the host of the virus life. The virus is the changer of the house your consciousness chose to live in while here on earth. Viruses change the boundaries of your physical outer biology and your biochemistry inner world. It's time we realize that our cell nucleus is of viral origin, so I believe. Therefore, instead of just trying to find a solution let's also try to dissolve the problem so in the future it is no longer alive.

The problem in our world today is two-fold;

One, how do we stop new viruses from entering our body. Two, once in the body, how do we dissolve or at least neutralize the environment inside our body so these predators move out and no longer find our bodies appetizing.

When a virus is completely assembled and becomes capable of infection scientists call this new and latest but not yet final version of the virus a virion. So again, the virus-virion has three parts.

The three part virion virus has the following qualities: 1) There is the inner nucleic acid core surrounded by the outer castings of proteins known as capsids. The Capsids protect viral nucleic acids from being chewed up and destroyed by special host cells enzymes called nucleases. 2) Then the killer virion gets the envelope. This final covering is derived from the previous cell membrane of the living host: 3) Then stolen bits of information are modified and used by the virus to allow the virus to continue to attack the other cells inside the host where the virus has taken up residence.

The primary role of a virus is to reproduce and survive by feeding on your life source. Your energy that makes your body work. Your energy is glucose. That is the substance that feeds our organs.

A simple definition of glucose is now needed. The word glucose comes from the Greek word for sweet (Glykos). But glucose is not sugar as society leads you to believe as it sells you its latest snake oil to allegedly help your diets and your health.

It is important that you hear this naked truth. Sugar is also broken down into glucose. Glucose is what your body uses for its energy. It's called blood glucose. Some scientists call it blood sugar. Insulin is a hormone that moves glucose from your blood into the cells for energy and storage.

Our living organs are what makes us work as they act in unison in a perfectly tuned vehicle, i.e., our body. However, our medical system with its partners, Big Pharma, in its health care for profit game isolates the organ when it gives you medicine to cure a particular ill without regard to what new ill this medicine will cause the rest of the balanced machine our body was created to be. And the sickest thing is we allow Big Pharma to advertise their latest snake oil on TV where the most people over the age of 35 sit and watch the sporting events or the news 24/7. In these commercials if you listen to the ads you are told in a different voice the damages this new chemical pill may cause to your other organs.

Back to viruses. For a virus to survive please visualize this simple truth. The virus needs to trespass your body and break into the inside of your body. How does the virus do this? Well the passages to get inside you are obvious. Those passages are the following: 1) you breathe it in or 2) you have an open passage which includes a wound and the virus gets inside your body through this passage.

Another way to get inside our bodies for the virus is using another invader. Who are these invaders? Invader one is the insects who bite us. These insects with their new virus give their hitchhiker virus the ability to take the passage from the insect to us via the bite as they have the mechanism in their

DNA or RNA to make the jump adjustment through the bite. This is how the disease we call Yellow Fever as well as Dengue Fever enters our body.

Another way into our body, is we bring it in knowingly or without questioning our imperial society by eating foods or drinking water that our system knows is contaminated and can make a new virus to join our world order.

Please hear this as you read this. We now eat food in the world not made by nature. Meaning it is not balanced for the ecosystem nature gave us to live in. This goes for the water we pollute as well as the air we breathe in our industrial profit first world. The world our imperial national governments support at the costs of human life. This changes our body and makes our organs in some cases not able to withstand the virus invasion of our body parts.

The job of any community government is to run the true economy of the community. We need to really, finally understand that economy is much more than chasing paper profits. A metaphysical economy is really learning how to live and maintain a balanced earth for the community of mankind living with nature, really Mother Earth's balance. It is not us, currently living, telling nature these are the changes we require you to accept.

We have mixed up truth. We believe and maintain that an economy is to fix the trade of materials or ideas as the reason a government exists as opposed to protecting the community of people the government was created to serve.

Economics of industrialization and urbanization of the Earth for personal profit business alone and the pursuit of accumulating currency from these businesses are the causes of our new viral diseases. And when I hear blue or red teams in the U.S. making regulations to limit, as opposed to stopping wrong behavior, I get sick. Because if it is poison, even a little is too much. We are changing the balance of our world. This is not climate change alone. This is world change. We are creating new life and with new life comes new viruses that run our RNA. And these viruses steal the DNA code information that gives us all life. And in doing so they change our lives.

But hear this too. Viruses like C19 make us indispensable as a whole to the virus. Therefore, it will kill the weak, but it will not kill most of us. The virus will just create a new human inner being, one that can live with this new virus. Now some of us, who are very aware and hid these truths that the food they sell us with GMOs both biological and chemical (such as Bill Gates who owns Monsanto now part of Bayer) will be investing in the cure to protect their clients from altered GMOs bodies.

The goal is to have the mass customer keep living off their privately owned food source, which seeds they privately own for personal profit. These new modified seeds or ingredients we put in our soil to make things grow create the environment for all living beings to become the experimental lab for new viruses unknown to earth. The FDA speaks with forked tongue as they are really the rubber stamp for GMOs and the industrial globalization when they proclaim these new seeds fit for life, they have not experimented with the full life and the effects these new seeds make over the lifetime of earth's subjects. They are paid to say yes.

Noun scientists say the virus is not alive but in fact a virus lives to reproduce and survive. It has no consciousness of what it is doing. It just does. But in naked truth we are all viruses as we are predators who must eat living organisms so we can change that food into glucose for us all to individually survive. Now I must repeat that sugar is not glucose. Sugar, like all foods, must be broken down to become glucose to run our bodies.

By making fake foods or chemical food without life force our bodies must continue to break down this new food into glucose. This new creation is the cause of Diabetes II, a new disease much different than Diabetes I.

We have now created a world that is the laboratory for new life called viruses to come and join new and stronger than before and bury themselves in our bodies looking for the glucose. These viruses go to the organs that are supposed to get the food from our metabolism that works to separate the glucose from the ingredients we put in our body.

I feel I must now share with you all a very simple truth, I have Type One Diabetes. Type One means I do not make insulin. So therefore, I must put insulin in my body for my body to take the glucose inside my blood and feed the cells as the blood is really our river system.

Hear this please. Diabetes Two means your insulin does not work the way it was made by your DNA to work. Our foods today hide the real glucose. Glucose is not sugar like we all think it is. Glucose is the substance that runs our machine. All food that has any life has glucose. But in the fake food the glucose is hidden. When the food is digested, which is GMO's fake Mother Earth food, it takes longer to break down the food to glucose. So, our bodies' minds are teased and our minds send signals to the body saying glucose is coming when it is not yet ready. Doing this makes our insulin make false runs to the blood assuming that blood is carrying the real glucose needed to feed our cells. This confusion in essence shuts down the system to dissolve your glucose as the body was made to do so in the first place.

Once you get Diabetes Type Two fat, your body's game plan does change. Your built-up fat delays the real feeding of energy your body needs to work as created to work. Your glucose ends up being peed out of your body and your machine stops working as intended. Your organs revolt and you get sick. So, this little supply of glucose that has found its way to the organs is a perfect place for the virus to attack because this is where the virus will get the energy it needs immediately. Healthy organs will fight off the virus most times. A healthy body is hard for the virus to enter and steal ingredients it needs to stay alive in your body with no other purpose than to stay alive. A weak organ does not have the strength to keep fighting the virus off as it tries to steal some of your glucose.

My point is the following - yes, we have a contagious virus that we must get the serum to kill. But until we stop with our profit at all costs for the industrial world, we will only be fighting new viruses that get into our body from the foods we eat, the air we breathe and the water we drink. As I told audiences around the globe, agriculture must not be an industrial machine. Earth decides what she grows to feed us. Every time we change this simple truth, we infect all living beings with new viruses.

So, we need to make changes in our lifestyles at the same time we put out the inner fire of the virus running alive in our bodies and attacking our weakest organs, which includes our respiratory system. How we allow tobacco companies to sell cigarettes laced with nicotine knowing it kills us shows us how predatory we are. We kill others knowingly. Monsanto type of businesses are just as guilty.

Many conventional scientists of history not practicing scientists who live to discover more, will disagree with this essay. But remember they feed off the system they were taught to perpetuate. This needs to end. And we need to start rewarding those few who have the nerve to stand tall and discover more than this is it. Unfortunately we do live in a paper profit bean counters world. So when we discover something is wrong, we hide the need to make changes accordingly, as these changes would change our paper-before-people economic stream. We hide the truth. And once in a blue moon we do try to fix the issue instead of dissolving the issue.

Our world Imperial Order of gods and their Imperial Government is profit before people.

This is vampire time. And yes, we are predators who need to eat life to stay alive, but we also have a consciousness where we can stop being predators as our way of Imperial Religion and Government life. We are not here to kill each other for sport and please know that business is really a sport. A fixed sport for the few to rule over you at that.

We, as a group known as mankind are here to help us all survive and thrive in a world that lives because one must be a predator. If we ate each other it would make more sense. But we kill and then bury the bodies, so the worms get their food.

In 1992 a team of researchers discovered a bacteria-like structure inside some amoeba which were living in a water-cooling tower. These scientists led by a man known as Wessner realized this was not bacteria but a very large virus which they called Mimivirus. The virus is about 3/4 the size of the then known smallest bacteria and was thought to have the same properties as the Gram-positive bacteria.

Gram-positive bacteria is the term used to describe scientists test of bacteria to figure out what they should do with this new form of life. Bacteria works both light and dark in our world of life. But know that what is dark for us is light for some other organisms that need those results that the bacteria cause to occur as it lives its bacteria existence.

Again, we need to account in truth for what we do to each other. Digging up fossil fuels and releasing long buried energies is opening a chasm of long buried fossil virus. Know that truth. As our glaciers continue to melt, frozen viruses will now come back alive. Viruses that I believe affected earlier forms of life before mankind became the top animal on the ladder of life. We are changing life at its simplest form.

How about fracking? And do know fracking is one of the causes of the newest gases released from earth by our invasion of earths natural order. Our government of the people allows private entities to blow up earth with dynamite so machines can trap the gas so released, as if it is a fart and bring that gas out to be exploited. How? We refine that gas and sell it so the few who run our industrial world can continue to profit at the expense of the health of our community. Maybe it's time that some true leaders, who cannot be bought, start implementing the change now from fossil fuels to solar energy.

We are poisoning our earth. So, we eat this poison in our food derived from this poisoned soil. The poison also gets into our water and poisons the food we eat from the waterways that gave us the food. Plus, the water we drink that we store in reservoirs is poisoned. The water is not pure. We drink it or the vegetables do and then we eat those vegetables or we eat the domestic animals who graze on the poison grass. But it's ok because we can now pay our bills with interest to third party bankers who graze off this continued insane behavior. The industrialization of Mother Earth's natural gifts so poisoned. Please know that when a product says it is "organically grown" it is still grown in that poisoned soil.

Since this is a stream of consciousness, I must now make you all aware that the FDA's of the world are as good as their intentions are to lie to us all. There is no way we can approve new foods and drugs until we see what it does to mankind over the span of man's life.

The burden of proof to prove the use of new drugs and food must be put on the applicant to show what it does to mankind and to the environment of all living beings over their lifespan. The burden must not be placed on those who contest the new energies i.e. product that the third party for profit is trying to put into the cycle of earthling's lives.

I hear you say as you read this, the scientists say the drugs, or the food is ok to ingest that the FDA is here to protect us. No, the FDA is here to authorize in our imperialistic business world order, the spreading of the new products into the commercial avenue and this game instead of protecting you the consumer, the FDA actually protects the maker of the product from lawsuits of willfully doing wrong. Now the excuse is we made a mistake. This difference is big in civil lawsuits liability.

Please note, that these scientists who authorize the use are part of the system. Each test the paid for scientist does is potentially rigged. We need to know what the change does to its flow over our lifetime. Not what it does to a mouse or monkey who has a shorter time to live. If we need a bandage to stay alive that is one thing but to use a bandage and not fix the problem that is another thing.

We need to stop the lies. And when our 44th President Obama brought a Monsanto lobbyist to run our FDA it made me sick. This man promised changes and all he did is tow the industrial world line. When the future generations look back at our time here on earth, we will be the idiots not a blue or red team member. We sold out for an industrial material way of life.

Bacteria vs. Viruses once loose in your body have different purposes. Bacteria has more than one purpose. Some bacteria are harmful, but most serve a useful metaphysical purpose. They support many forms of life. Bacteria are microscopic, single celled organisms that exist in the millions in every environment both inside and outside all living organisms. The bacteria that causes colds in mankind eats our glucose not the sugars we eat. The bacteria need the real glucose. So to kill the bacteria disease you starve it. Different than how to kill a virus living in your bodies organs.

Viruses serve no purpose but to find an organism that it can invade and then infect and direct the cell machinery to produce more identical viruses for the virus community to live in this infected organism. So, it may make sense that a human must be fit so the virus cannot find a weak organ to latch onto and infect that body because it found the weakest organ in that body. Meaning, do not starve the infected body glucose. The one infected must eat. The organs must be strong.

Let's move on and review chemical warfare. What is this? When did it begin? Is this not the birth of a world that has given us today Covid 19?

Chemical warfare is defined as using the toxic properties of chemical substances to kill, injure or incapacitate an enemy. Our accepted Science Daily report claims that we, called mankind, have used at least 70 different chemicals in the last century to kill each other.

What about this century? Are we not killing with chemicals using new foods, fracking and just all forms of our industrial world that polluted the waters, the air and land? Is this not chemical warfare against earth by mankind?

But back to the last century. Let's look at the birth of the Spanish Flu. And discover her makers

What is the Spanish Flu? Why Spanish? This flu was called Spanish but not because of its origins. The flu then was caused by H1N1 influenza. (yes, that one). The flu traveled the world from the Fall of 1917, when the world was experimenting with germ and chemical warfare as those governments killing each other trying hard to make their new world order. That flu lasted from fall of 1917 till the summer of 1919 we are taught but that is not true as we shall see.

In the interim the flu hit and entered the human bodies of, reportedly, 33% of the world's population. A population which was estimated at 1.5 billion. So, 500 million got infected and ten percent meaning 50 million plus people died.

When you research the Spanish Flu, the Chinese get the blame in some reports, but no one dares suggest it was caused by the World War I participating governments and their industrial killing machines' new way of war. It was straight up a new way to kill.

Those killing chemicals were released into the air. This is the first war using airplanes. In the air the weakened war bodies inhale the chemicals and those bodies got infected. The soldiers returning to their families infected their communities too. Also, please be aware these chemicals affected our plants and animals which includes birds located where the chemicals were tested as well as released in the air as I said and now by plane.

They say in our history books that a vaccine stopped the continued spread of this flu. However, at the time the flu first hit there were no vaccinations for this flu. And the vaccinations the people created were for the wrong virus as the Spanish Flu was a novel virus.

The virus was also said to have started with birds which then got to us humans. The first public announcement of this disease was in the US when a military man in Kansas was diagnosed with this new disease that then had no name. It was later called the Spanish Flu because Spain was neutral in World War I which was really the world war family feud between Queen Victoria's Grandchildren and their three imperial kingdoms' Russia, Germany and the UK. By the way all three believing in a form of Jesus Christ.

So, historians today still called this the Spanish flu because Spain, being neutral, was the only country at that time reporting the new flu. But do now that Spain was involved in many wars during the years that led up to World War I. The other World War I nations were withholding this information for as long as they could because they were at war and they needed to concentrate on killing the enemy. This flu was everywhere.

Soldiers traveling in and to communities around the world nevertheless had the distribution network to get the newest manmade disease.

One historical view is that the US was the spread of this flu. The U.S. entered this world war late and our soldiers went to France bringing this bird disease and it spread around Europe. However, I have a more global view. Chemicals made new life and that new life affected all beings living here on earth.

Countries fighting the World War I withheld knowledge of this disease from their pop culture media world. Spain, not being involved, told the truth. But like C19 the Spanish Flu was novel.

There were no vaccines for the flu as I just said. But also, there was no known antibiotics to treat the secondary bacterial infections. Then, as now during the beginning of this pandemic, they were limited to non-pharmaceutical solutions such as isolation, quarantine, disinfectants and limited public gatherings. Now we have vaccines coming. Great so now you get a shot and all of a sudden the virus is dead. Damage done and so we can continue our polluting ways.

Reviewing history, the first flu vaccine to be licensed in the U.S. was 1940. So, in 1919 this Spanish flu just had to run its course. It did we are told. But it was an influenza.

C19 was at first thought to be a chronic acute pneumonia. Which means it works on your breathing. It's not chronic acute pneumonia and we are now understanding that this is a new Coronavirus. This C19 probably existed before December 2019 but did not have the mass exposure it does now.

This is a new breed. We need to deal with this truth. We need to kill the ways diseases feed on and off us as well as how and where they enter our bodies and attack the cells that will feed the virus the glucose it seeks.

I will soon give you the physical exercises we must all do to raise our energy levels so we can stop the virus at its port of entry. We need to strengthen our bodies and that means changing lifestyles and our current capitalistic industrial military complex that searches the earth looking for new limited warfare all for its profits.

We need to admit things change. When things change, we must change our individual as well as collective behavior. We cannot continue to do what we know is wrong behavior. This is true no matter what the initial intentions of our behavior were.

Let's look at Polio.

What is Polio? Polio is a virus that causes paralysis. We are told it is prevented by vaccine. But once in the body is not able to be cured. Polio spreads through water and food. Polio came to light when our industrial world order started dumping chemicals into water on a large scale. This virus got its fire to exist in water polluted by the chemicals of mankind.

Let's examine other viruses over the life of mankind of our written history world.

Let's call this section a quick summary of the social history of viruses.

Let's start around 13,000 years ago when mankind lived in what we call the Neolithic period. The Neolithic period refers to when mankind became civilized and really urbanized. Instead of being hunters and gathers we became machines to exist for the imperial gods and their governments.

Civilized really means domesticated so those who were part of an urban center worshipped the gods that spoke to the rulers and their priests to keep the people in line. Give them their food so they can be the slaves to the urban rulers in other ways now that they are being fed mass industrial foods.

This is the beginning of the industrialization of mankind. This was not a worldwide event. There were many people living then living with nature. In the history books they were called pagans. They knew nature and they understood they were part of nature. Urban centers created a concept where those who lived in those centers, pledged their allegiance to a Father God and forgot Mother Earth. And they believed it was ok to destroy Mother Earth because Father God you were told by the few said it's ok.

This way of urban life was created by organisms who came to colonize earth and created mankind. We know of these organisms as the gods who came from Nibiru and are also known as the Nifilim. These gods created mankind by creating the seeds and wombs of beings and planting those seeds and eggs inside a womb with the characteristics of animals that lived then on earth. The Nifilim are mentioned throughout the Old Testament, as well as, specifically, in Genesis 6:1-4. The word Nifilim is also spelled Nefilim if you are now looking it up. Different spellings cause confusion. Look for the energy of the word you seek.

These new mankind creatures needed to be civilized to serve the few gods and their royal retinue, so they needed grains and other foods not present, here on earth. So the Nifilim brought the food in both plant and animal form. This created a new environment where the gods lived and with this new environment came new viruses to feed off the new living plants and animals now serving the Nifilim and their slaves or servants called mankind.

Know this truth, Mankind has 233 new enzymes that first appeared on earth when mankind miraculously just appeared about 300,000 earth years ago. When you research and discover this truth you find that we are told these enzymes just appear and get transferred to the new apes, our founding fathers and mothers by bacteria. Bacteria we are taught infect the new beings and making a horizontal transfer of information for both the DNA and RNA of the beings we are told were apes.

Plus note, our consciousness is not from earth. We live in a body we borrowed from earth to perform services here on earth as an explorer on a mission. Now we have no mission, so we need to discover and accept that our bodies work on earth's laws not what we wish for but regulated by earth's laws. Mother Earth is our body's boss.

So, with new and improved livestock and agriculture, now our way of urban life, we acquired the viruses that live in and off what we eat. That simple. Look up potyvirus of plants and/or rinderpest of cattle and other even toed mammals. It's mankind's history, the creation and spreading of new diseases. We change the environment and nature creates a new virus as nature tries to rebalance what we are doing to nature's world.

Two of the oldest viruses known to mankind are smallpox and measles. First, they lived in animals who eat certain plants. Then the virus jumped to us. This began in lands of urban agriculture in the old Middle East and Europe.

When the Vatican conquistadors invaded their New World, those invaders brought those diseases to this side of our globe. The Europeans had their immunities to these diseases, but the natives of the new world did not. This is really the beginning of intentional germ warfare. Then germ warfare was the newest game and was used to conquer and control these new lands for the Europeans to mine and destroy.

Sharing diseases was not one-sided. The Conquistadors came without women to steal for the imperial King of Spain and their Imperial Religion called the Catholic Church. As they did not have brothels to have their sexual releases they would rape the native women and apparently have sex with both the cows and sheep of those territories.

These conquering heroes on Columbus' ships in 1492 returned to their homes in Europe with Syphilis according to the new skeleton evidence our explorers have dug up. When these killers brought their stolen booty to the Vatican cities in 1493 and 1494 the new disease was introduced to Europe as the new virus dance. The first well recorded outbreak of what is known as Syphilis occurred in 1495 amongst the French troops and their Spanish mercenaries besieging Naples, Italy. By 1600 this disease had spread to London as well as Moscow. Surprise, surprise, each government blamed the other.

The more we change the environment the more we give space for a new virus to come and make havoc. We tried to make life better for us without regard for the balance earth had before our change. New lineup makes a different team.

I love history and even though it is fixed and does not represent the true picture as it is often a one-sided view in the true, naked story. I still learn from the lies to discover what they try to hide in plain view.

A true historian, like a true scientist is really a verb. A true historian, questions everything. And since the facts that contradict the story are hidden you must learn to feel things with intuition and then let your intuition lead you to the true story of why things happen the way they happen. Doing this you will discover who are the puppets and who are the puppet masters?

We can feel truth emerge as we learn to question what that one side view is all about. So, let's go through time and learn about viruses and how imperial urban mankind tried to cure them even before we in this era knew what a virus or bacteria were.

Let's visit the land today we call Egypt

There was a ruler named Siptah during the 19th dynasty, who lived around 1292 to 1189 BC. There is this Egyptian Ancient Stela that experts believe shows signs of a poliovirus victim. See the picture in the photo I section of this book. This is the first pictorial sign of a virus we call polio.

Then during the rule of Rameses V (20th dynasty) explorers examining mummies buried during that time 3000 years ago our experts claim to have found signs of smallpox. The living humans then had no idea what was what. So, they created gods to worship to heal bodies inflicted with the latest virus disease.

Let's move on down the linear road of mankind called time till 430 BC. Let's zero in on Athens. A war nation we call the birth of democracy. This imperial regime went to war with the eastern part of their world. They were not merchants like the Romans they were just warriors to kill for their King. When the warriors came home from the invasion of todays Middle East all of a sudden new diseases began to appear.

One of these new diseases was Smallpox. We are taught smallpox wiped out maybe 25% of the Greek's tribal army. Plus when the conquering heroes came home they infected the so called citizens and their slaves of the city of imperial conquest again which we are taught is the home of democracy. But democracy for who? Remember this democracy had slaves of all colors.

Now on our globe visit of the past let's visit the land once called Babylon now called Persia. Let's hone in on the era around nine hundred years later after the birth of Jesus. Now here we can learn of a physician named Muhammad ibn Zakariya al-Razi. Long name right?

This Muslim first identified what we today call measles in our recorded history of mankind. Remember the Vatican who controlled Western Europe did not allow anyone but their priests to read let alone write. They had all the answers and if you questioned their story you were a heretic and removed from society. This is the history of the Ashkenazi Jews after Genghis Khan moved them from Central Asia steppes into Byzantine Eastern Europe. Another story. Another time.

Dr. Rhazes called the disease Hasbah. It came from domestic animals of this urban region. This disease was our measles. A measles infection if you survive it confers lifelong immunity. Therefore, this is key, this virus requires a high population with density to become endemic. Endemic means the infection is maintained and does not kill the hosts it is found inside. The virus has found a place to live and live off as the hosts do not die.

The measles virus had been around since domestic animals came to earth and started feeding off the grass that was now created. This era again goes back to what we call the Neolithic era, the New Stone Age when farming first appeared here on earth. Really when somehow mankind started altering life forms then living here on earth. How did we do this? It's in my book Collinization of Earth. Another story. But the point here is new viruses appear when we alter what's on earth for our purposes alone. Not to keep the balance of earth the way that earth wants it to be.

Measles in Egypt back then was not considered a disease. No, it was a stage of development or a test the child with the help of some new god would survive.

Let's go to what we call the Middle Ages. Europe has humans mass reproducing. Urban centers meaning dense populations are on the rise. This population explosion based on the urbanization of farming is ripe for viruses to jump from animals to mankind and I must add to start new life inside us in the first place.

Animals had rabies. You have heard the term rabid dog I am sure. Or bats with rabies? What is rabies? Rabies is a contagious and fatal viral disease of dogs and other mammals with digestive systems similar to mankind. The virus feeds on glucose and glucose travels to your blood before it reaches your organs to feed off your living machines separate ports of group machinery that make our body run.

Plants use the energy of the sun to change water and carbon dioxide into glucose. Glucose is used by plants for energy as well as to make cellulose and starch. Cellulose is used to build cell walls. Starch is stored in plant seeds as well as other plant parts. That's why mankind and other animals eat the fruits and other parts of the plants. We get glucose from the plants. This is the true partnership of life here on earth. We give the plants the carbon dioxide.

Rabies causes madness, convulsions, transmitted through the bite and the saliva the bite transmits when it bites a new living object.

I experienced rabies shots when my Artist decided to bite the head off a bat while on stage in Des Moines Iowa back in early 1980's. Ozzy, the artist was trying to find his path to his quest to become the prince of darkness. He succeeded to a degree. My role was then to get him on the road after his arrest by allowing the authorities of Des Moines to release the artist from their jail and to do so we had to agree that the performer was to be shot with twelve rabies shots around his stomach as if it was a clock. And do know Ozzy survived this staged event of his and it is today part of the folk lore of rock and roll history.

Not everyone died from rabies before vaccination. But many did.

During the later middle ages, a new disease invades Europe. This epidemic was the Black Death. Black Death was not a virus but bacteria.

Bacteria as we have discovered are single cell living organisms. They have a cell wall and have all the DNA components to survive and reproduce. Bacteria does derive from other sources. Those sources are viruses, so I believe.

And as we have read scientists are arguing whether or not a virus is a living thing because to survive, the virus must hitchhike a ride to exist inside with another organism. A virus must find a host cell to survive long term and get the energy called glucose to live and reproduce.

My belief, again, is all life here on earth began as a virus. The virus is consciousness. This consciousness started living in the forming atmosphere that surrounds our earth. Earth was created from the gasses which the sun's energy was changing into material substance of both earth a solid and water a living liquid.

I must put in right here that all life starts as a gas. A virus searching for a body to call home. With energy we call fire, the gas called by me a virus can be alchemized into a liquid or a solid or both. A gas is airborne. In the air the sun gives it life.

Once you have the water, a virus living in the water and getting the energy from the sun creates bacteria and that bacteria creates more bacteria and soon you have a team of living and breathing, reproducing cells. And these cells grow. The cells can become plants and then fish and then develop the organs needed to create reptiles and mammals living here on earth.

My belief. I see it as I write it to you. Also, this is how life began after the words "Let there be light", according to the Old Testament. Light is energy, which I call consciousness, looking for the physical spot or to create the spot to land and then live. Think about this truth.

Black Death was the worst pandemic recorded in our human history timeline. Took out between 75-200 million people during its run here on earth. Did it die out? Or did it survive with herd immunity? Who really knows as all life mutates to survive meaning the bacteria figured out how far it can go on living in our bodies.

Where did this begin? No one knows but my hypothesis is the following: the Vatican cities called the Vatican states back then controlled the Western European travel to and from China as the traders traveled to entered the Asian continent. The Imperial versions of Christ were successful in keeping the Islamic Imperial Religion who controlled our Middle East out of Europe until this disease hits.

I believe the travel to and from China or the other ports in Asia had rats that carried this black death bacteria. We are taught about Marco Polo as the man who discovered China. All crap. The Vatican controlled the trade routes to Europe and there were many seafaring men who did this travel and dumped their wares in today's Italy as well as the Balkans and North African regions. And yes, there was land trading too on the path we call the Silk Road. And it was more than the Vatican's myth of their hero Marco Polo. The Vatican creates these myths as they need to own those great daredevils who risked their lives for mankind to acquire or discover more than what already exists. And there is so much more than this. That's why the Vatican made one character the central figure when they are really explaining a way of life by those who lived during that character's era.

So back then the Black Death era, the rats carried fleas from their regions and these rats took a ride on the merchant ships leaving ports and coming to the Mediterranean regions. This includes North Africa. These rats now living in these new regions attract fleas. Fleas bite and take on your blood as they need the glucose carried inside your blood. The blood of all mammals. New fleas attack the rats and get the Dracula blood and while staying alive bite humans too. Guess what?

Now humans are infected with this new bacterium, for the first time and we have a" new viral infection" trying to find if mankind can host this bacterium called Yersinia Pestis.

The Black Death disease peaks in Europe in our timeline around 1350 AD. Look at the changes in the world of mankind back then. The Vatican lost many of its living constituencies and the European dark ages is about to end. The Islamic imperial killers tried to take over the Balkans. The Chinese Imperial Naval Order introduced the printing press to Europe around 1434.

The Western white world that our European descendants live in of the Imperial religion called the Catholic Churh is about to begin to be questioned as unconditional faith was not the answer. So new myths are created and written to perpetuate the role of this Imperial Christ. This is also when the Jews became the alleged carriers of the Black Death and had to be removed from society of Europe. But not entirely as the Catholic Church needed "a them" so they could have "an us".

Viruses and bacteria need to survive. They will find herd immunity by trial and error. Unfortunately, C19 is in its trial and error period. The weak will be attacked and those strong enough to survive will survive for the most part as but do know our bodies have a limited warranty on earth life in the first place.

There's another plague I have just discovered that I must share with you readers. The Plague of Justinian.

Who was Justinian?

Justinian was the last Roman Emperor as opposed to Byzantine Emperor. Justinian was based in Constantinople around our time we call 527-565 AD. This man shut down the Eastern European Schools of Sacred Knowledge. He really started the European dark ages. The school then taught you metaphysical life, love and how to prepare yourself for the afterlife when your body dies.

But if you are the current living boss, of the Christian Imperial God created by Constantine and his bishops who created catholic awareness back in 325 AD says so, the game of control requires you to limit knowledge to only those who will perpetuate your regime. The new intellectual caste system.

Justinian is also known for building churches and bridges. He made dams and built forts to keep out the viruses of other mankind's thoughts contaminating bodies and getting the bodies to kill for who and what is god.

In fact, this man rebuilt the Hagia Sophia. A beautiful cathedral in today's Istanbul.

But there is another story of this Imperial Regime so lets call it the Plague of Justinian. The Roman Church was still one Empire. The boss was housed in Constantinople. The city was created by Constantine, the creator of the myth we call the Catholic Church. It was created to justify Imperial Roman rule. And this rule had to move to Constantinople so the rule could control Europe and the Middle East as well as North Africa.

So now in 541 AD a pandemic hit this region known as the Eastern Roman Empire as well as the Sassanian Empire of Persia and the port cities of the Mediterranean Sea. The Sassanian Empire was the last Persian Empire before Islam took over. And Islam which took hold in 622 AD was perpetuated around this region from this epidemic.

That epidemic which fossils confirm, was caused by the Bacteria called Yersinia Pestis. The same as the later Black Death. Authorities claim this epidemic took out 25-100 million earthlings. But that was over two centuries.

What this plague did do is destroy the exclusive ruling order of Eastern Rome in this region. It also allowed the Pope and his Cardinals living in Rome to create their own rule of intellectuals called the Vatican. This Vatican needed its own army and this army they created is the First Reich or the Holy Roman Empire. The First Reich that ruled Europe with the Vatican appointed Queens and Kings in various lands which Empire Napoleon ended on his run (in 1806) to be the new living god.

I have read that archeologists found this bacteria strain of this era in the mountain ranges we call Tian Shan. Those mountains exist in today's Kyrgyzstan, Kazakhstan as well as China. They claimed this discovery means the Black Death started there. In fact, the whole species it is also claimed of this bacterium can be traced back to Qinghai China. I believed this as the Chinese have always experimented with ways to increase yields of agriculture plantations on their lands.

Qinghai China is a landlocked province in the northwest of China. The disease started in the people's agriculture and farming region of this area. By the way, today's Wuhan, the alleged birth of C19, is not far from this region then called Qinghai. What does this mean? Ask the experts. But again do be aware that this region does create new ways to make more food per square foot than before. Which means new chemicals being introduced to the soil.

Now to the Renaissance era. Around 1500 AD. Our country today we call England not yet Great Britain beats the French at the Battle of Bosworth on the European continent. The date line is 22 August 1485. Henry Tudor is King of these Brits invading other lands to control trade and get their Value Added Tax as these winning nations guaranteed to the losers safety if you paid for their protection. The real history of Imperial War.

As the victors were now eating produce from lands unknown to their body's birth digestive system, the English troops came down with a disease called the English Sweat. Or maybe the French mercenaries themselves who fought for England brought it back to England, but somehow it did infect the British on their land of our world.

By 1508 the new disease was affecting England differently as it hit mostly the affluent who ate differently than the masses. The rich would eat different parts of the domestic animals that were raised to feed the people. The rich were poisoning themselves with luxury.

That summer of 1508 was unseasonably hot for London. The disease spread and victims died within 24 hours it is so written. The streets were deserted except for carts carrying dead bodies. King Henry VII declared the streets of London off limits except for physicians and apothecaries. This King, the first Tudor King dies from this disease and his 17 year old son become the infamous King Henry VIII

The trail of this disease then surfaces in Hamburg, a big trading port with the English. Even in our time period this is where the Beatles went to perfect their trade before their invasion of the world. The invasion was based on harmonies with songs based on love in the 1960's.

History says 1 to 2 thousand died each week in this northern water European border town called Hamburg. Hamburg then was a free trade port. Meaning no tax to any church or church government. The disease spread to the rest of a region we then called Prussia and then Central Europe all part of the then Holy Roman Empire. Do note there was no nation called Germany till 1871 after the Franco-Prussian War. The name Germany comes from the word Germania which has a Latin root. Julius Caesar may have actually coined the term the "germs" when he called them germen referring to the tribal people living in that northern region. The Latin word germen means seed or sprout.

Historians bet this was a flu. And a flu even today does take out many people each year, but we are ok with that because today we have a flu shot and Tamiflu. We believe that makes us safe from the influenza. Influenza is a Latin word meaning influence. Derived from earlier Latin word, influere, which means to flow in.

And I must add all these terms have Latin roots because in Europe of the Western Empirical Church only the few who joined the first communist party I call the Vatican were taught how to read and write. And they were taught Latin so the Vatican believed they could control the virus of knowledge. Fortunately, the virus of knowledge has spread into many different languages. The only alternative back then on the European Continent was Greek. If it's Greek, it comes from the Eastern Byzantine Church.

Medicine was not yet a science. So those in control did not know what to do so they blamed "the them" in their society. Who is "them"? Them were the Jews and other tribes who somehow got into their Vatican lands. These outsiders were soon banned. Travel restricted was implemented. Stricken families were quarantined. These families were isolated from their communities. Buildings were set on fire and livestock were killed.

The Isle of Hispaniola in our Caribbean suffered an epidemic after the Vatican's conquistadors arrived to colonize the natives with their Vatican lies. The source of the disease was pigs. A swine flu did its work. The Europeans had herd immunity so eating the pig did not kill them and the natives who had no pig before were killed off.

The Europeans also brought the flu and measles as well as smallpox to the new Vatican or Christian conquered territories. The Europeans brought back venereal diseases that had herd immunity for the natives in their Native American territories. These conquistadors infected their white European communities with these diseases when they returned home.

Viruses are everywhere. And again, all life starts as a virus. So, I believe. I repeat everywhere. .

Luckily, Europe had the brave few who questioned the Vatican when searching for answers. An Italian living in the Vatican States named Girolamo Fracastoro around 1500 AD thought and then tried to prove measles was spread by seeds spread from person to person. Conceptually a virus is really a seed that gets into us through ingestion or air. So, he wasn't wrong in the metaphysical truths of the universe. The man did write his study of Syphilis which is the birth of Epidemiology.

Let's visit London which had Agriculture plagues in 1593, 1603, 1625,1636, and 1665. This in our story called history is today called the second plague pandemic. The pandemics did fizzle out after taking a huge proportion of the English and North Sea area as well as English Channel population.

I must remind all of us that true farming practices from ancient knowledge teaches us farmers not to consistently use the same soil year after year with the same seed. We need to rotate our crops. These rotation rules were broken when the population exploded and we needed wheat or potatoes to feed the masses. Really a starch. The soil stopped working and we created new ways to impregnate earth with the seeds. We created our own viruses and new disease.

Now England in 1670 with its own church which was unlike the Papacy, had a church that instigated others to become aware as long as the English Crown which was also the boss of the church got their piece of your economic pie, had a new nation wide virus. They called it an epidemic. One of their doctors named Thomas Sydenham said this disease is caused by toxins. Vapors coming from earth. You are taught he was wrong but maybe those toxins were none other than virus released into the air by the farming practices the English Imperial governments were using making food to feed the masses.

Some more epidemics for us to read about and I begin this section with the Yellow Fever. A disease, we humans get by mosquitoes, the Yellow Fever first appeared 3,000 mankind earth years ago.

This Yellow Fever caused trouble for the European conquering heroes making their new world order. Thieves maybe the better word for these imperial conquistadors. It's 1647 and we are on the island we call Barbados. John Winthrop an English Puritan lawyer is the governor for the then Charles I of England in the last years of Charles's rule.

This lawyer passed the first ever quarantine laws in North America. The quarantine did not work. It did not work because the disease was coming from the economic trade amongst diverse populations. And the economic trade was more important than a few lives.

But understanding trade amongst diverse populations brings disease from other regions. You can stop viruses from happening in the first place. We live in earth's bodies. So we need to stop contaminating the Earth. We need to know that truth.

So how do we survive Covid 19 today and then get community herd immunity or at least the antibodies that will help us survive till then?

How do we stop this never ending crisis?

We stay healthy. We eat healthy. We exercise. We create governments that do not disrupt our ecosystem and balance here on earth. We stop Monsanto's and others from making chemical GMOs. We stop digging fossil fuels or blowing up earth to trap gasses. We stop polluting our waters with toxins that the fools in our government regulate believing it will reduce the harm. Harm is harm. Get it! We had better.

Just for an aside let's discuss how humans kill plants by spreading disease with the things we do for love or prosperity.

Once upon a time in the 1620's the seafaring Dutch brought the tulips back from today's nation we call Turkey, then the Imperial Ottoman Empire. These tulips were unique and quite a joy to behold in the darkened European cities. You plant the tulip in the fall, before the winter freeze and early spring your area is blossoming with the colors of love the plants give to share. Share with all life I must add. Not just share with mankind.

These tulips were the must have pet possession of that era. And it then became a stock market scam. Bet on what color these seeds would bring to you was the gamble. Look it up under Tulips. Great story.

Now in Dutch paintings of that era you can see striped colors on these tulips. Today we learn that these stripes were caused by a plant virus. Humans gave the plants this virus from using jasmine in the soil to help the seeds grow. Jasmine grows in the warm temperate regions of Eurasia and Oceania. But not in the Dutch lands. This meant that future tulips would not be guaranteed the stripes that made the plant so beautiful and special.

How about the potatoes of Britain and Ireland as well as Europe? Remember the famine that got Europeans to come to America because their food was not growing. It was called the Great Irish Famine. The era is 1845-1852 in Ireland. But there was the famine in England fifty years earlier. And people moved to our Northern America contingent to eat starch that they were now able to grow again. The potato disease was not the mold found on potatoes that caused the blight. No, it was a virus called the Potato Leaf Roll Virus.

Point is viruses are everywhere. And all life is subjected to our earth changing ways. Get used to it. Stop panicking. Stop being divide by your god or your political party. It is time that mankind in this Age of Aquarius shares openly information that concerns the health and welfare of all mankind. When disease hits, when we mankind become aware, when we see it, we must share information freely world-wide. Or else the latest virus will continue until we get herd immunity.

Just as a reminder, that some of us had lived through these industrial agricultural pandemics. Let's look at the 1957-1958, Asian Flu pandemic. This was a global pandemic of influenza, a virus now subtype H2N2 that originated in Guizhiu, China. China, where the nation had to figure out how to make more grains and starch to feed its exploding people population. When you want more food produced from earth than earth is capable at that moment of producing, you must change the constitution of the soil. This change creates new lives which I call viruses. By the way, it is estimated that 1.1 million people died worldwide during those two years.

Now let's look at 1968. We had the pandemic which was caused by Influenza A (H3N2) virus comprised of two genes from an avian influenza A virus, including a new H3 Hemagglutinin, but also contained the N2 Neuraminidase from the 1957 H2N2 virus. This virus first appeared in the U.S.

Let's look at the 1997 Hong Kong Flu. It is written that 18 people were infected and 6 died when H5N1 bird flu first jumped the species barrier from poultry to people. In late December that year, the governments ordered the slaughter of 1.3 million chickens in a bid to stop the spread of this virus disease.

No one will sit and try to analyze how the poultry got the flu in the first place. These diseases to earth's living inhabitants are 100% caused by mankind's industrial urbanization of agriculture and our urbanization of the waters, land, the seas and the air. We need to be aware.

Let's move to the History of Vaccinations.

Where shall we begin?

Remember I was school trained to think European Christian Order before the world. My educated school knowledge has the Vatican and their imperial lies and distortions of truths as my base. As a child going to the programmed schools of 1950's and 1960's America I was not allowed to know that there was another educated and enlightened world. Not one living elsewhere in the dark Vatican ages.

I say this because I have discovered as I am researching that those alive in today's Turkey, again the Islamic Ottoman Turk Imperial Empire, had a local practice called Variolation and today we call it inoculation. This method actually began in China long before the Renaissance era of Europe. And the Ottomans and China did share information.

The European Renaissance is really when the Chinese Imperial Navy landed in today's Italy around 1434 and gave the Vatican City States the books they called Britannia, with records of how the Chinese created their great society. These books told one how to make a printing press. Taught one how to make noodles and pizza plus so much more. They told you how to plant food. How to grow produce and feed animals.

It changed our then white man's world. It also had maps of the what the Vatican calls the New World where the Chinese and other pre-Colombian cultures had been living for eons. The word Peru is a Chinese word that means misty. The coast of that southern land region, Peru, is misty. When you sail in from the Pacific, which by the way, Balboa did not discover, the coast was veiled in mist.

The Chinese vaccination process was simple to learn but we did not have schools of sacred knowledge let alone any schools of any form of higher knowledge as a way of life in that European Vatican era. That is unless you were becoming a priest with ambition to be a bishop and even a cardinal. And if you got that high maybe even pope. But to go up this ladder you needed to keep secret your knowledge of the way earth works as you were now part of earth's controlled Imperial Religion and its resulting European land order run by Vatican approved Kings and Queens and their royal retinue.

So the Chinese and the Islam regions used a process to immunize an individual against a disease spreading from new victim to new victim that was not yet part of your bodies knowledge on what to do with this virus to kill it or let it continue to feed off you.

This is how those then did it.

Someone other than the victim aka patient, would take material from an infected human being or animal and put that material inside another human being or animal. This was done to stop the spread of the disease in man or animals. How did they do this before shots?

Here are the smallpox cures back then. The party administering the cure would insert or rub powered smallpox scabs or fluid from pustules into what we call superficial scratches they made into the skin of the one who is going to be cured.

Now the patient with these scabs would develop pustules identical to those caused by the naturally occurring smallpox. This means the disease has entered into the new body and this dosage would infect the patient with the disease but not as bad.

Then two to three weeks later those symptoms subside and all would hail out loud the patient is cured. This was used in the White Europe world under protest in the 1720's. But it is how the idea of vaccinations began. We need a safer method was the cry. And the few who explore and know there is more than this go out and prove it.

Before I continue to take you through the history of vaccines, I must introduce you to the reasons for children's nursery rhymes and really fairy tales too. Because in the lands of Catholic Imperial religion rules you were not able to question the Vatican's position on why things are the way they are. You just had to listen and believe.

Faith was the Vatican command and our Christ who died because of your future sins would save you only by following what we tell you to do. Truth is if you question the rules you too would die on the cross. So those with awareness communicated in riddles for children they say.

Really these rhymes labeled for children were the rap songs of that era. The songs gave you hidden truths in the prose of these rhymes.

Do you know the Ring Around a Rosy rhyme? Do you know how and why it began? You will now.

The rhyme is Ring a Ring o' Roses,
A pocket full of posies,
A-tishoo! A-tishoo
We all fall down.

Ok so this means what you now ask. Well back in medieval England, where this rhyme begins, a rosy was a rash. The rash was a symptom of the plague of death. Posies of herbs were carried as protection to ward off the smell of the diseases which your sneeze would keep you from inhaling the disease into your body.

This was the advice town leaders would give each other so as not to offend society with remedies the Vatican did not own. The Vatican actually told people if you die god wants it that way. The Vatican could never share the naked truth. And that truth is Father God is not in control of Mother Earth's pantry which we call also a womb.

In the 1760's men in the land called the United Kingdom started preaching that a cowpox shot into the arm of a human could cure smallpox. Cowpox was a disease that those who touched the uterus of a cow to milk the cow would get the signature cowpox pustules on their hands.

By 1796 a doctor named Edward Jenner vaccinated James Philip, then a boy with the first UK vaccination to stop smallpox. This proved in time to be the remedy.

Variolation was soon to end with the new method called vaccination. Interestingly to me is that Russia then in 1805 became the First Nation to outlaw this Variolation procedure.

Variolation may be said to be done in our world but it still goes on when parents have children's parties trying to share the newest community infection. These parties were called pox parties. A pox party is where children were put together and intentionally exposed to diseases like Chickenpox, Measles and Rubella. Public health officials cry out this is wrong but the practice in our world still goes on. The theory is that kids can get better quicker than an adult and with ease survived the virus.

The word Vaccination comes from the Latin word vaccinus. Vaccinus is an Latin adjective and it means of or relating to cows. This word is based on the word vacca the Latin noun meaning cow. The cowpox material used for injections was then called vaccine. The injection itself got the name vaccination.

Britain in 1840 freely vaccinated the poor. Something we in the United States should learn to do. Living health care as a form of private capitalism behavior is wrong and so against Jesus and all his preaching. But Imperial Capitalism with Christ as its head needs to see and understand the harm this game commits to those who live under this archaic, immoral, unjust system. And if you have a moment realize that Jesus of love is not the same energy of Christ the enforcer.

Capitalism is for third party private profit. Health and Welfare must not be for private profit as a starting point. Please know that the word capitalism was never used until 1854 when it was put in a German novel called the Newcomes. Please understand that Adam Smith the alleged god of Christian capitalism taught that the wealth of a nation is the people of the nation. The people of the nation need to have moral sentiments which is the title of the book that made him famous in 1780's. He was not a private party capitalist. He was a man of and for the people. He believed that a healthy community of people would create wealth for themselves as well as wealth for the community. The Theory of Moral Sentiments.

Viruses and Bacteria Metaphysical Truths.

What comes first bacteria or a virus? Here is when we humans started to get the true picture of creation.

Back in 1900 the physical indisputable evidence of the existence of a virus was obtained. So, the scientist who can only confirm what they see which limits their ability to really cure now can say yes viruses do exist. The scientist then had experiments with filters that had pores too small for bacteria to pass through. So, the organism that filtered through these pores was then termed a filterable virus. Again we had microscopes finally that allowed scientists, to see the small vibrational particles which are not solid themselves.

Scientists then believed a virus was a small bacterium. In 1931 with the invention of the electron microscope scientists started believing that viruses were a collection of toxins. That is until they learned that viruses have RNA and some even have DNA.

Now we need to learn that some things are created totally out of gases that appear in our air. The alchemy of metaphysical truths. We need to learn to explore and hopefully accept this truth. And our industrial world makes gases for our lifestyle. Those gases, as said before, in the air come alive with the energy that the sun gives it. With this sun energy the gas takes on a new form be it liquid or material. Yes, life is created out of nothing. It begins as a gas. Learn that truth and our gases make the newest and latest airborne diseases. Not just for mankind but for animals, fishes and all plant life.

We need to wake up. Stop believing what everyone does as conventional wisdom. A scientist must work to learn and discover more. All life starts as a virus and viruses modifies and changes life as we know it.

If we want to maintain life as it is then we need to stop our wrong behavior. Not with regulations to allow some wrong behavior. No. Stop the behavior. Unless as a common species, we the community of mankind agree we will bear the risk of new life and an altered planet. If we want to stop altering our planet then we must agree to prevent what happens and we must share information. It cannot be privately owned.

Anything for the benefit of Mankind as a common community must be owned by all nations. That information must be public domain.

So, my solution at this point of time regarding C19.

One, we must share information that each nation learns without any hesitation. We must all agree that this is paramount to our race surviving. If not, we will make ourselves extinct. The rest of the living world may be better for our extinction but then where do we (the consciousness) go from earth. And yes, I believe in the afterlife as well as reincarnation. You don't die. Your body does not either. For when we leave our bodies and move on, the body starts decomposing and goes back into the circle of living earth. We become food for other lives.

Two, we need to comfort our citizens by telling the truth, which includes saying we do not know. We need to end the profiteers who own companies, private companies whose sole purpose is to profit by controlling the knowledge of our physical life. This includes those few who have patents on our genes. All needs to be nationalized. Immediately.

Three, we need to print and put in circulation the money needed to keep our health active and alive. Watching blue vs red arguing if the individual states or the U.S. Federal government should pay the bill makes me sick.

We print money. Let's print the money needed to give us health. And while we are at it, let's end the Federal Reserve as a private, third-party for profit, system. We need to control our national central bank. We need to wake up. The bank is an asset of the government and we must understand the government is an asset of we the people. When this is not true, we need to do exactly what the Declaration of Independence said. We then need to create a new government. One that is for the people, of the people and run by the people so to be governed. This truth is not a third-party corporate scam organization that puts businesses privately run and privately owned in front of the people by bribing those two political parties with funds to run for office and be their puppets. The game called Political Payola. For a moment, please reflect on the Big Corporations that sponsor political campaigns as well as their political conventions. Same puppet masters who rob us blind and give their puppets a few crumbs to do their bidding.

I ran for Senate and Congress here in the U.S. to help our people. I may be crazy because I know and am very aware of too many things. I ask questions and demand answers. Plus, I investigate everything I hear especially if I realize this information is not truthful as it is only what I need to know so the person sharing the info stays in control.

My personal opinion, educated and backed with indisputable facts, is that this C19 disease is manmade. It comes from our sick and demented lifestyle where we believe we can ruin the balance of our air and water and land both above and below.

A vaccination will not end the Viruses. The gases we produce with our industrial urban lifestyle must end. If not we are only a moment away from the newest gases that Earth spits out of her womb from our polluting ways.

We argue about climate change and even there our leaders' solution is not to act right now but many years in the future. Got to keep my puppet masters happy is this crazy theme. We need to wake up! We change the balance of earth each day. And that change does not have a replay. We cannot go back. And we assume that earth will listen to us instead of remembering our consciousness may not be from Earth but our physical bodies are and Mother Earth controls our physical bodies.

We need home test strips immediately. We need our government to pay for it. We need to end the quarantine of no socializing outside immediately. Again immediately. If you are at risk stay home but free your families as the air you breath in your air conditioned or heated abode keeps the disease inside. And sooner or later you will inhale it.

You need to go outside. You need a health care system without insurance of private third parties profit before people. One that plans ahead. The monies are paid for out of the money supply our nation prints and gives to the Fed to circulate by lending it back to us. This is really the best gangster game ever.

I have spent twelve years of my life trying to educate our nation. Life is a communal sport. We must govern our lives as a community not with an imperial central figure telling us how we all must live. Each of us must learn to live in the community we currently live in. A nation is made up of many ecosystems, all different. One central force cannot rule these communities as if they are all the same. We may have similarities, but each ecosystem is unique and those of us who live in them must be in control.

Now let's take a pause as we move to how individuals can help themselves.

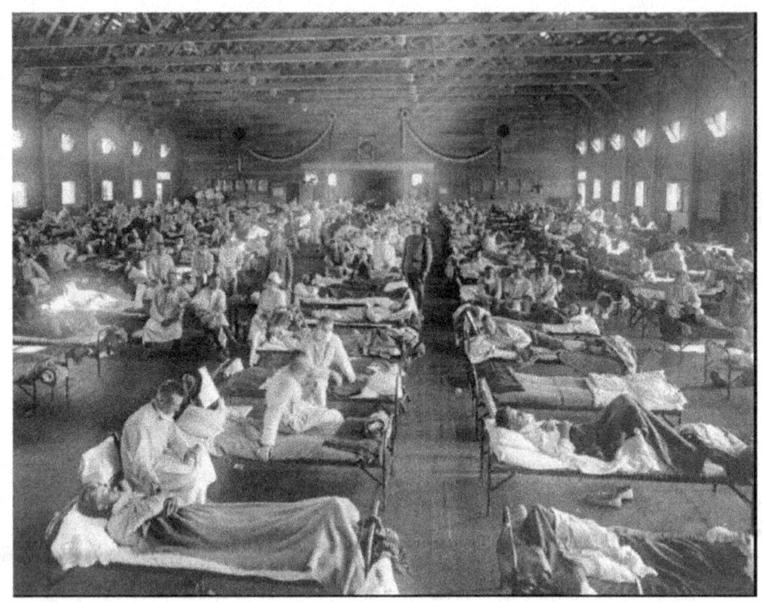

Spanish flu beds set up in a military bunker.

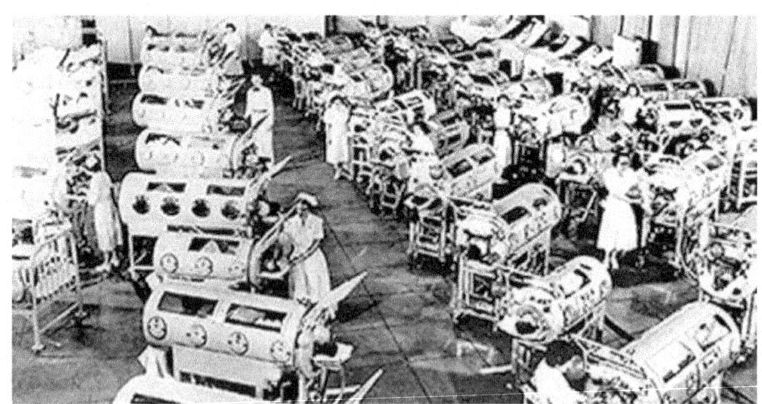

Iron lungs in the same bunker for polio victims decades later.

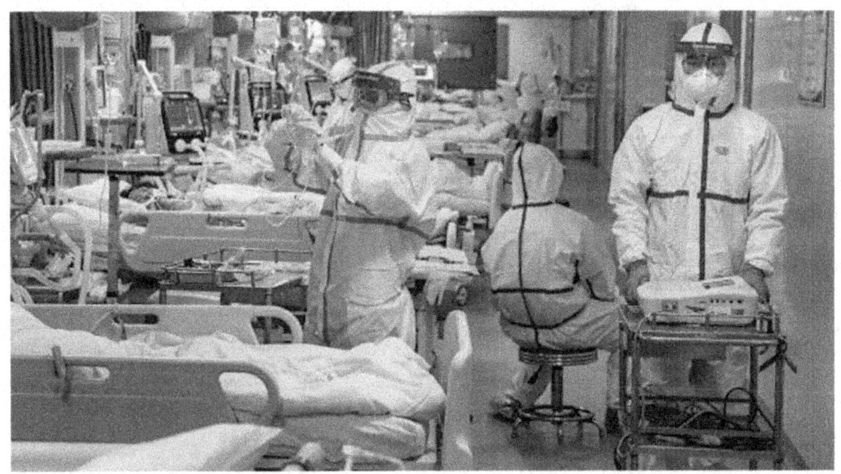

Over-crowded hospitals with Coronavirus wards.

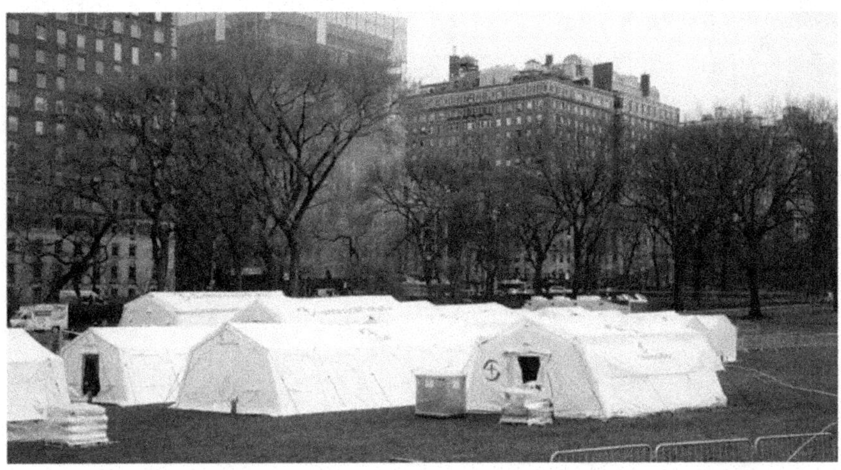

New York Coronavirus tents set up in Central Park.

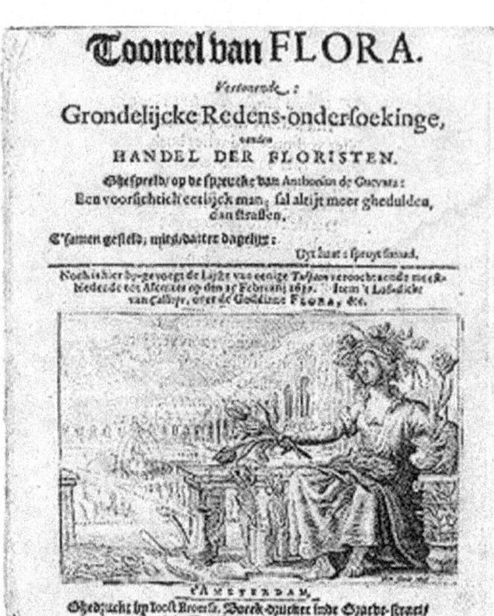

Girolamo Fracastoro
was a Venetian
physician,
poet, and scholar in
mathematics, geography
and astronomy.

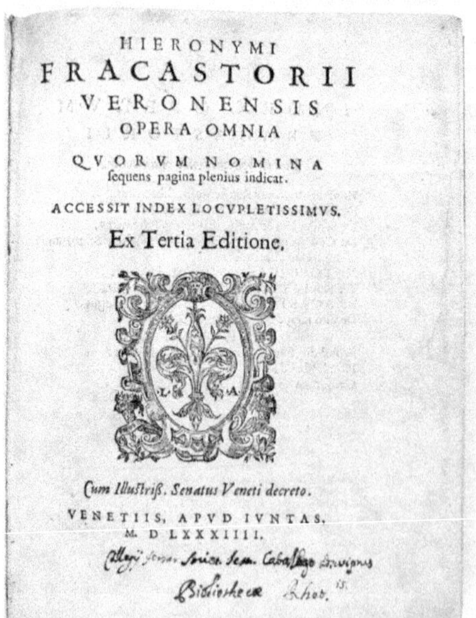

Fracastoro subscribed
to the philosophy of
atomism, and rejected
appeals to hidden
causes in scientific
investigation.
His studies of the
mode of syphilis
transmission are an
early example of
epidemiology.

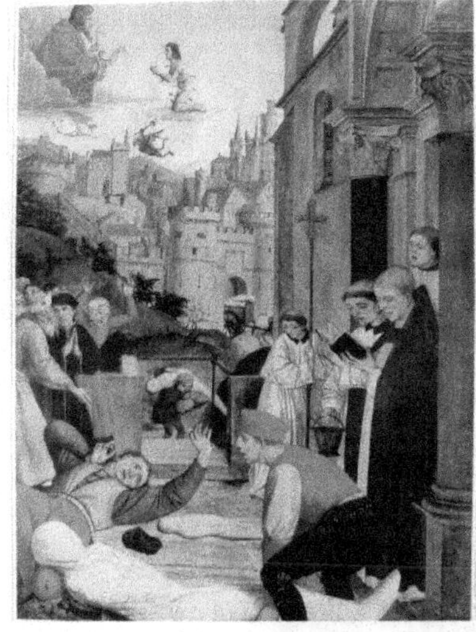

Plague of Justinian times.

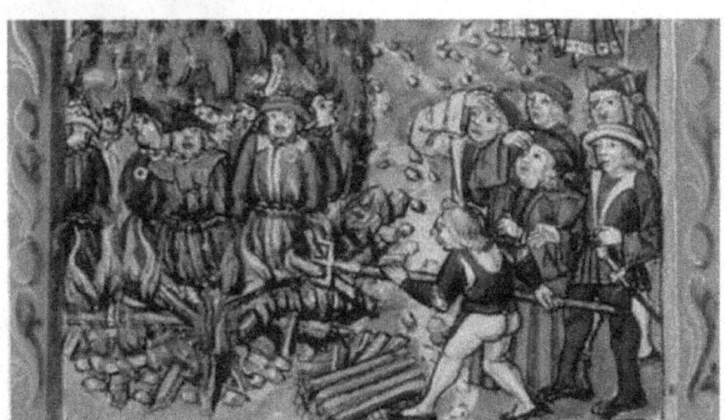

Plagues of Black Death. Church could not stop it.

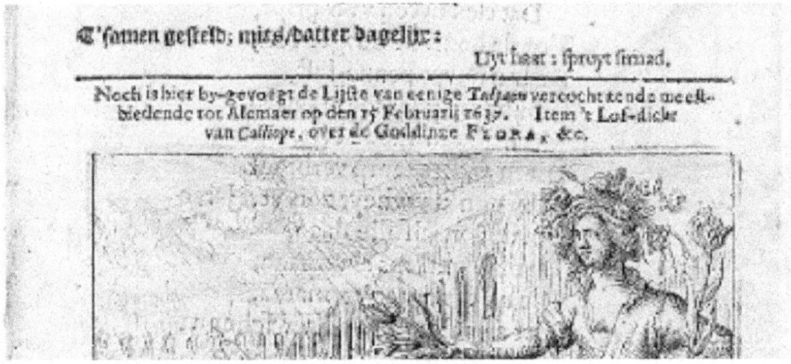

The sweating disease that swept through England 500 years ago.

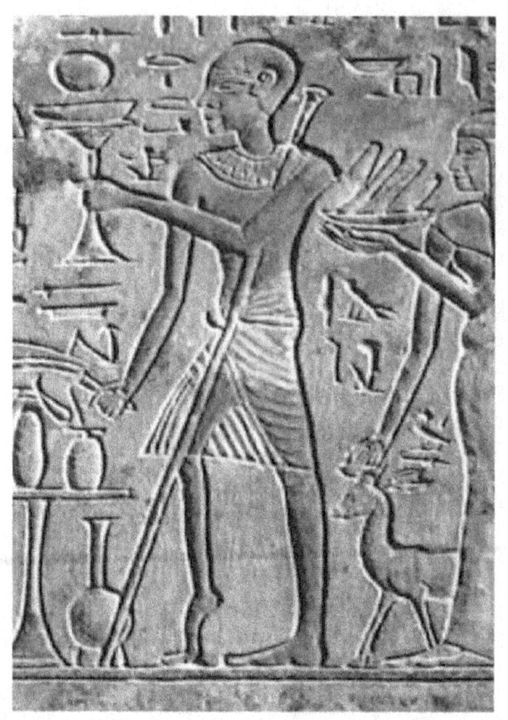

Example of polio back in ancient Egyptian times.
Back when grains were introduce to the Egyptian soil.

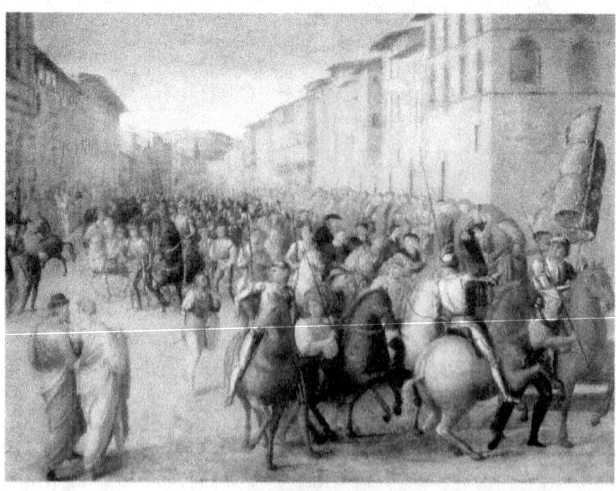

Medical upheaval due to the Black Plague.

Friedrich Miescher

- Began working with white blood cells in 1869.

- White blood cells are a major component of pus in infections. As a result, Miescher collected a lot of pus from bandages at a local hospital.

- Added a weak alkaline solution to the white blood cells– when he did the cells decomposed and caused the nuclei to move out of the solution.

- From the nuclei, Miescher isolated a substance known as "nuclein"

- After chemical analysis, nuclein was later renamed as DNA.

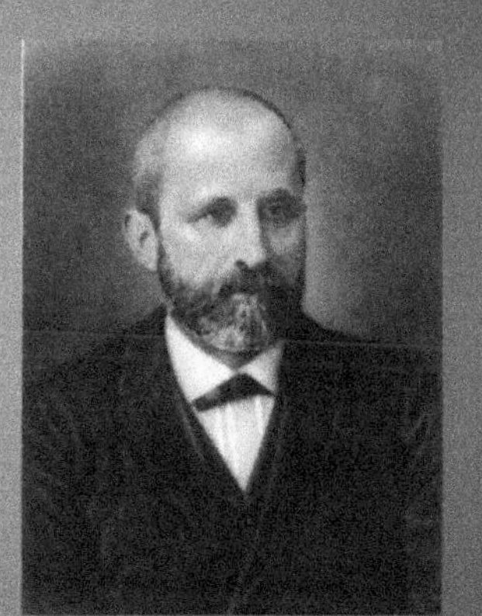

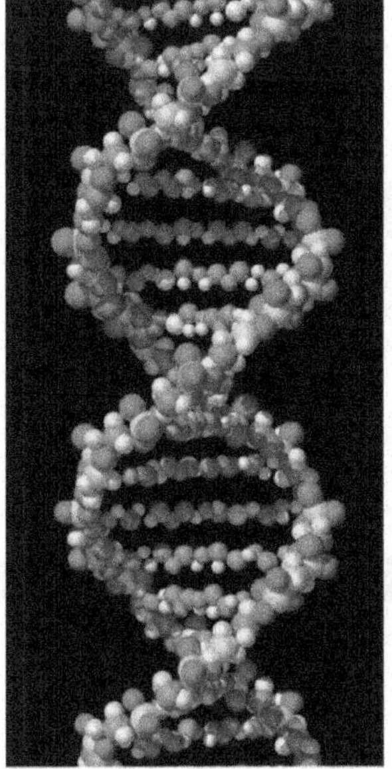

DNA and RNA structure

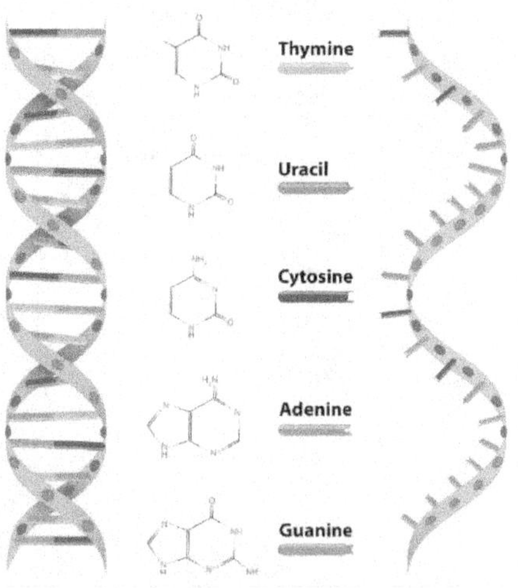

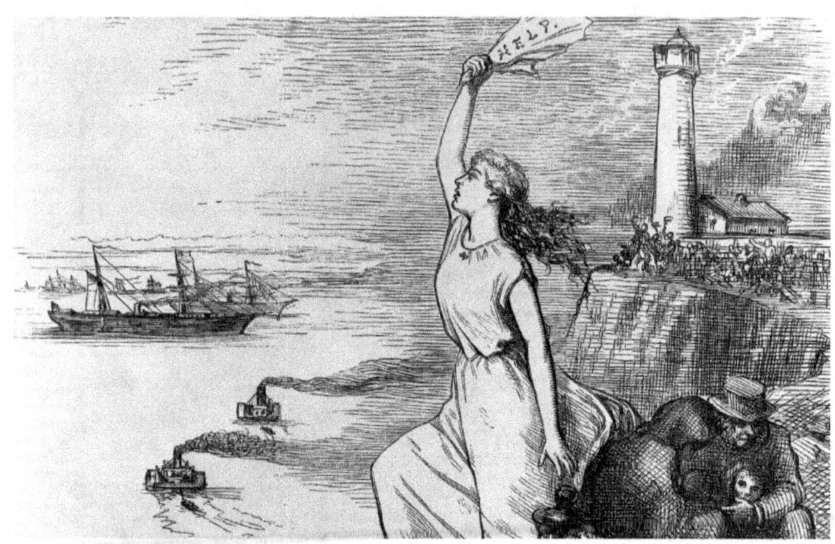

The Irish Potato Famine.

Muhammad Ibn Zakariya Al-Razi

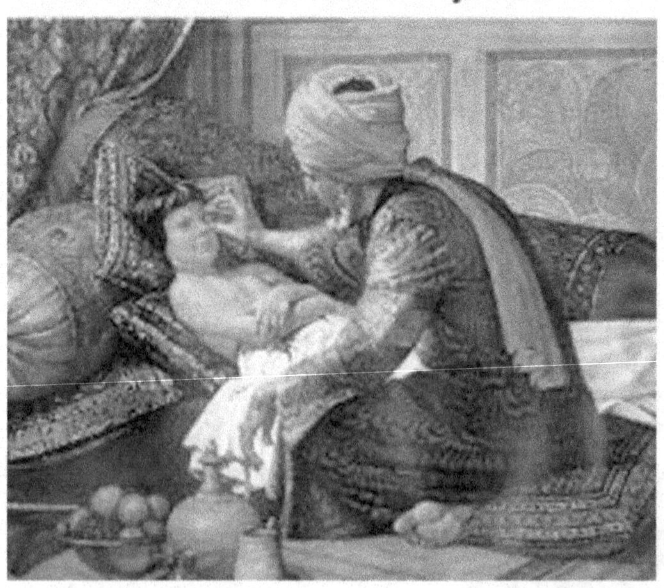

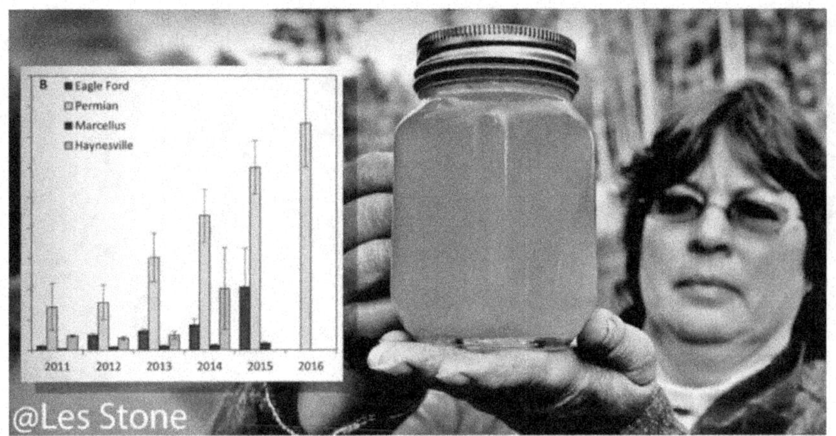

Drinking water after fracking.

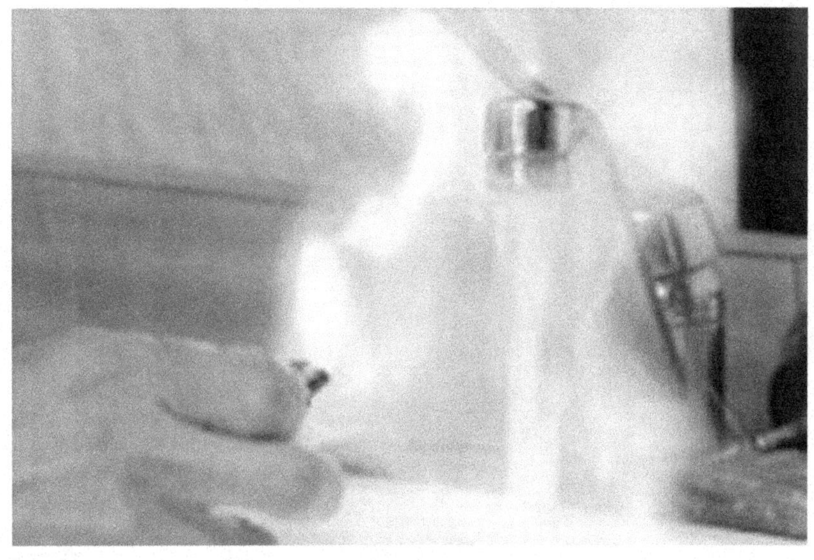

Flaming water after fracking.

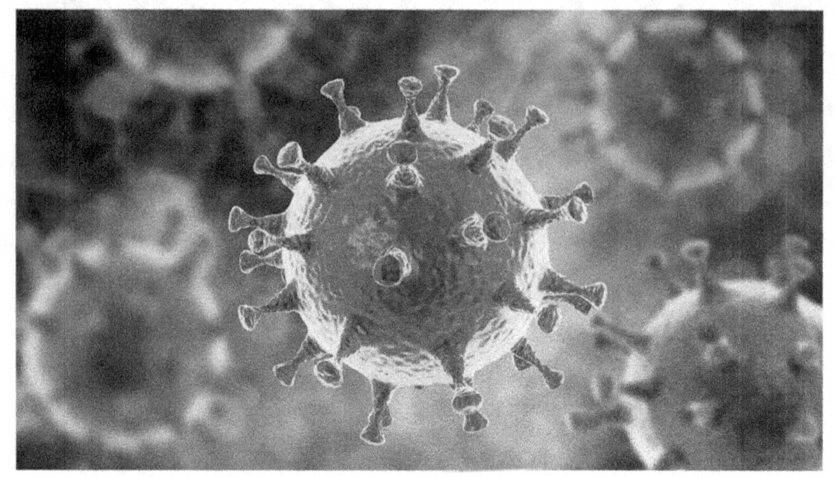

Coronavirus family portrait.

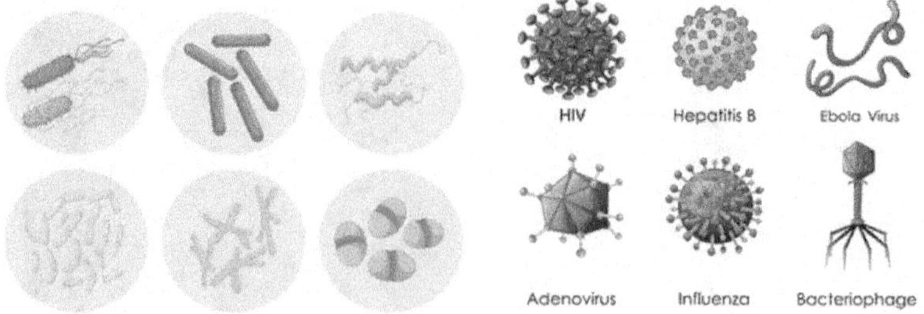

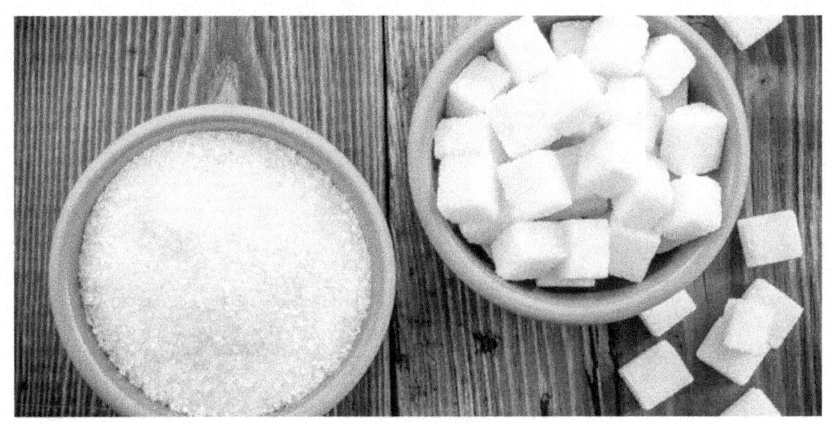

glucose

fructose

sucrose

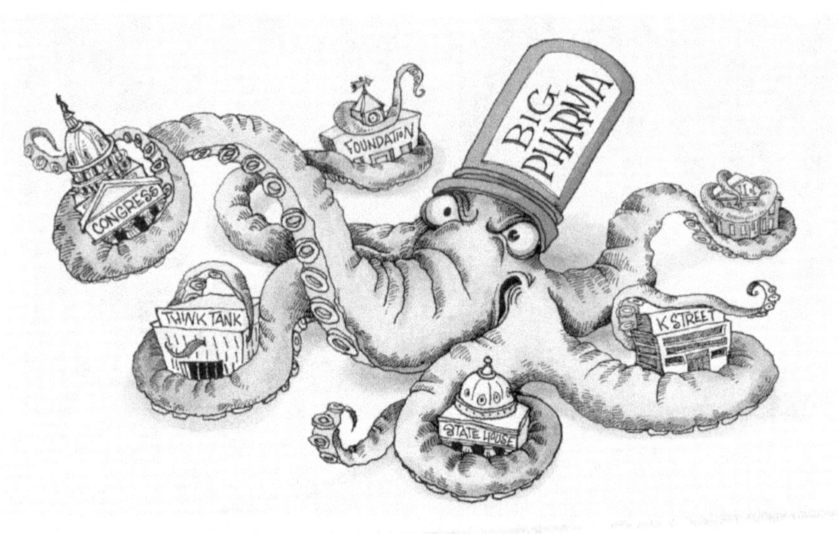

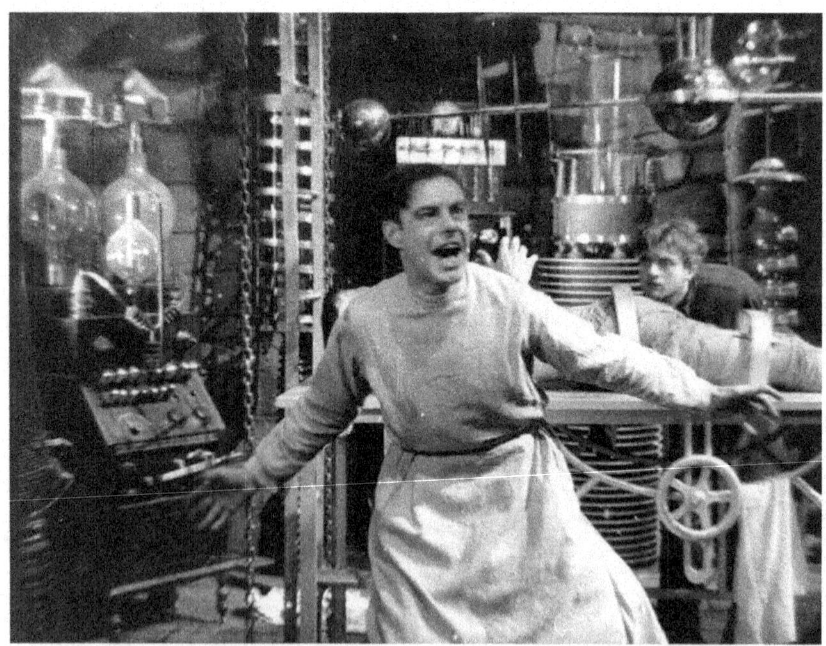

GMO scientist at work. For Franklin stein.

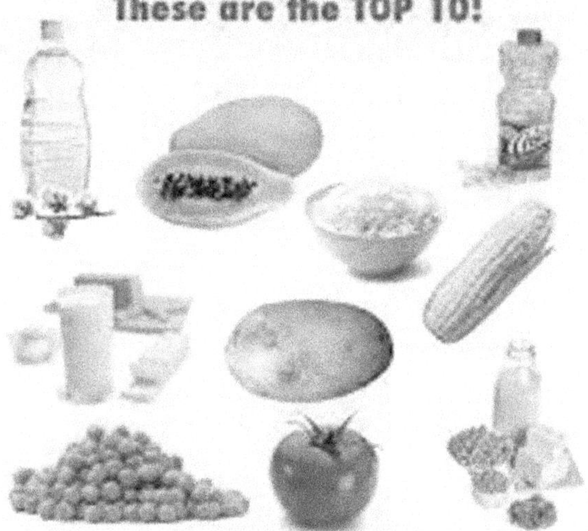

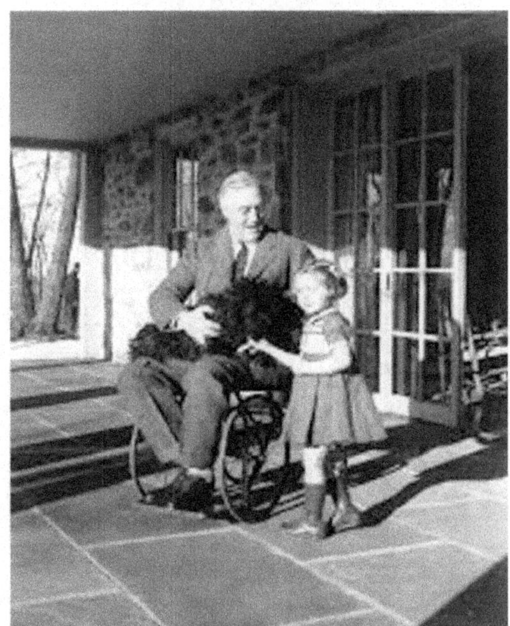

Picture of FDR. With polio.

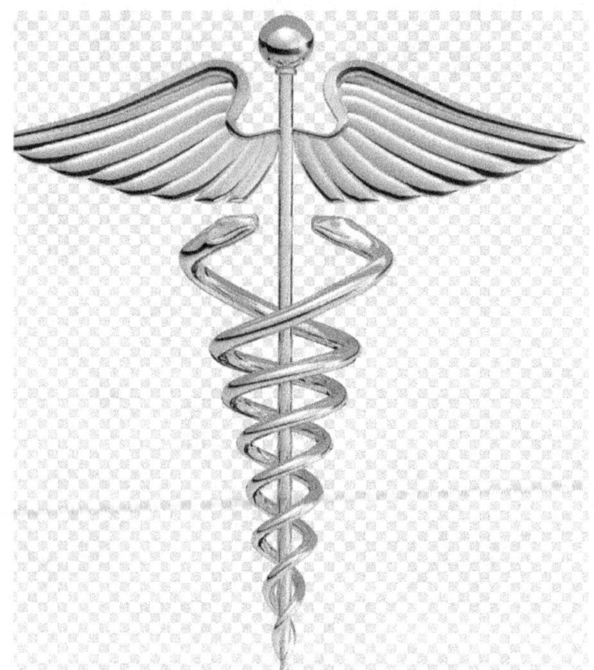

A physician's symbol comes from the caduceus staff with two serpents.

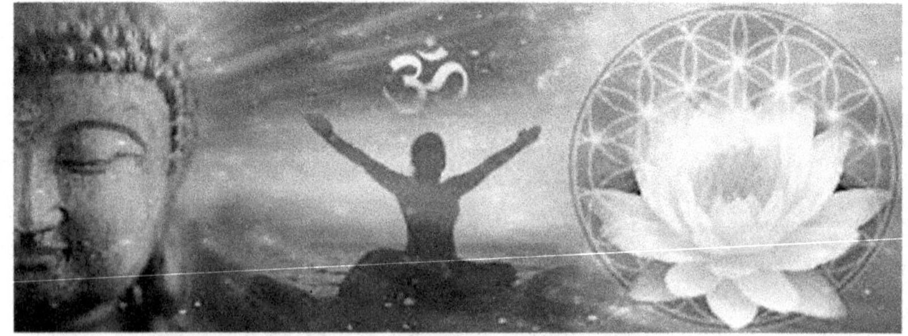

From thought comes life. The lotus is worshipped by those who are aware of this truth. The lotus grows seeking the light.

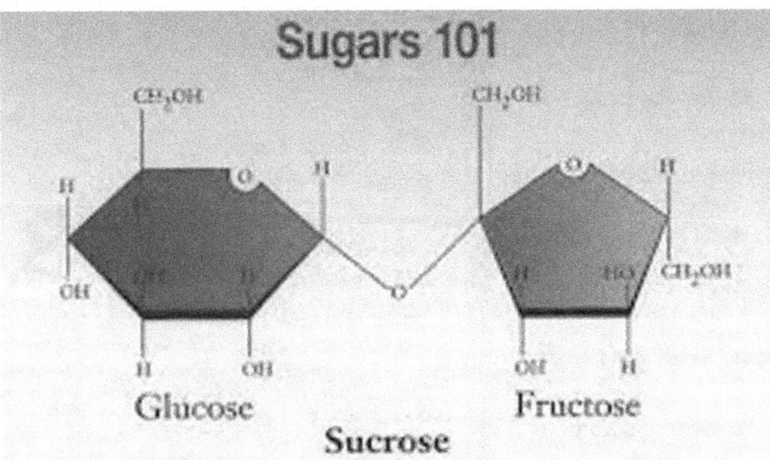

Sucrose (table sugar) is broken down—in the body and (to some extent) in foods—to half fructose and half glucose. At that point it is essentially identical to high-fructose corn syrup.

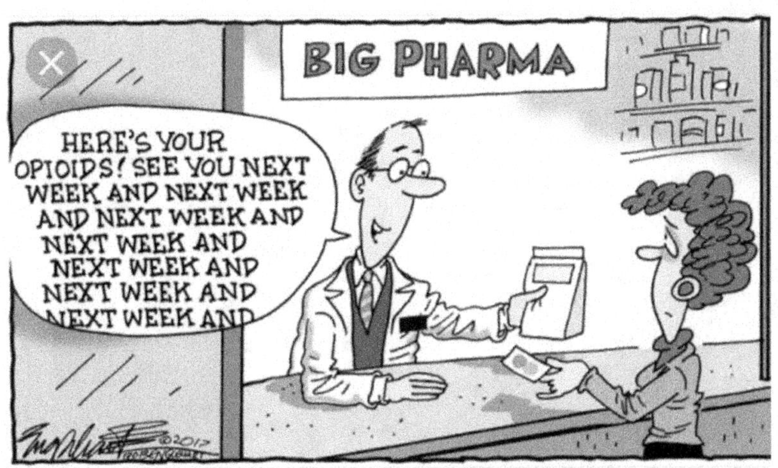

Part Two

How do we help ourselves?

Let's start with understanding what this tres-passer of our bodies is looking to obtain from our insides.

What happens when the virus enters our body?

This is what I can gather as of today from the research I have done. This is to give you an idea of talking points if you ever need to deal with the disease for yourself or your loved one's. I am not a licensed doctor and make no recommendations nor give any solutions except to tell you go to a medical professional.

However, we all must be informed of real possibilities which a centralized authoritarian figure does not like as it requires personal attention to the individual as opposed to group doctoring. Please note I write everything around the theme that we come from one consciousness but inside our bodies we are unique, special and healthcare requires attention to our uniqueness.

The facts, my friends, and nothing but the facts as of December 7, 2020.

People get infected by C19 it is believed, solely by breathing in the virus. The virus is the SARS-COV-2, which causes COVID 19. We breathe in the particles of this virus, the conventional wisdom says, in tiny liquid droplets, invisible to our senses in the air, and those droplets contain the virus particles.

Once inside our noses and mouths, professionals believe the virus attaches and starts to reproduce itself. Now here at this stage our immune system can do two things. The immune system may smell or feel the invaders and stop the assault. This first line of defense is what will stop the invasion for most of us. However, if our system is off the virus can do so much damage that the immune system is tilted like a pinball game and the virus can continue its wild toad ride inside our body.

Next stop, is our lungs. The virus sits in the lungs waiting room while waiting for the trip to our organs where the virus will feed off our organs. The virus' goal is to live with you inside your organs. The virus, while waiting in your lungs to get its blood boat ride to your organs does damage your lungs. When the virus first got the public's attention it was assumed that this virus was like the previous SARS virus. However, we learned that C19 has a longer shelf life to get to your organs.

If your lungs are compromised for genetic or lifestyle reasons such as smoking cigarettes the lungs will get damaged and this damage could be deadly. Damaged lungs from the virus? The lungs according to a Doctor Rainer Claus in the bodies of ten autopsied humans back in April of this year at the University Medical center Augsburg, Germany says that these bodies had lungs so damaged that it was impossible to see how any oxygen could navigate its way through them and do what oxygen has to do to make a body work.

So those are the entry ports of our virus according to the experts today. When you continue this investigation of truths we learn that the disease is actually not understood. Not enough time has gone by. There are questions without proven answers. Proven to be true over time.

Examples of how uncertainty plays the role of what do we do?

The virus C19 robs some of us of the ability to use our sense of smell thereby preventing our nerve endings to detect the invasion of our body parts. The doctors have reported the loss of smell as well as taste due to the virus entering our noses or mouths. We know this but what do we do with this information? Do we create a measurement that we can use at home to detect a new living entity upsetting the balance of our bodies function? Please be aware that the original C19 test was in fact, a sample taken from the back of the throat or nose.

Now with this information, what do we do? Do we invest in killing these droplets before they take up residency in our bodies? At this point they are only in the passageways of our bodies.

Let's continue.

In some infected patients the toes or fingers are dark, sort of bruised as if they hit something. Blood under the nails of the fingers or toes too. Blood clots will suddenly appear.

Hearts will swell in size. Not a good thing to have happen without the exercise that does make it happen. I was a serious distance runner and my heart did get bigger. A virus making the heart large by invading it, is dangerous as your body expands from external inputs not related to aerobics.

The question we now must ask is how does the virus get into our blood system and then our organs. The answer will follow. However, the remedy to Covid-19 is different than it was when it was in our respiratory system. This truth is what cost many deaths. And it was not intentional. We were blind-sided as a society to give proper healthcare and we are still blind-sided as the U.S. nation I love believes in insurance and not healthcare.

Now let me continue.

Covid-19 may in some cases just cripple our immune system. Then this crippled immune system can cripple our body organs from this invasion of the C19 body snatchers - the systems that the immune system is supposed to correct. This I believe is due to the fact that these systems are compromised as I discuss in this book. As I do believe the virus is looking for a private long-term lease of our organs to share not to kill us. The virus is looking for some body that can handle this virus load and stay alive as the new kid in town. Again, I must give you a caveat; this will not happen to most of us as we do not yet have a compromised system that cannot stop the invasion. This happens when we get old or due to our lifestyle.

But if C19 is in your blood you are now an experiment. Can John or Jane Doe survive the invasion? This C19 invasion is caused by our wrongful ways of living and treating earth as if we can tell earth what can and cannot exist.

What our scientists for mankind are looking to discover as the days of 2020 go by is how does this disease get put to permanent sleep or at least rest so we can take care of the damage it does to those who survive death plus to prevent deaths in the first place.

How does a virus attack the cell? How does it get into our blood?

Well the attack begins when the virus lands on a cell surface. It wants to get inside. To do so, the virus must be adorned with a protein. This protein plays a role in the regulation of our blood pressure. It causes inflammation and that inflammation of the blood pressure is called angiotensin-converting enzyme 2 (ACE2).

What is the protein that allows the virus to get into the cell?

We are studying the proteins of the crown called protein spikes. These are the keys that the virus uses to get into our cells.

These spike proteins of C19 are 80 percent identical to the SAR-COV, the parent of our new baby C19 virus. Studies suggest that the 20 percent difference is where these proteins got the ability to bind to our cells more so then the first SAR-COV. This is virus adaptation which we call evolution.

Remember that these spikes attack our weak organs. The organs that do not have the strength to know the invaders have invaded. They get through the first line of our bodies defense. The virus to survive needs us to be strong enough to survive the attack. So those with weak organs must be aware that the virus doesn't want to kill them. As we discussed a virus is a consciousness that wants your body to survive. It does not immediately kill you. It is hoping your body figures out how to stay alive so that C19 can also stay alive. But as we shall learn the lifestyles that many of us at this stage of the invasion have will not allow that to happen.

I will now continue the body invasion of this C19.

The ACE2 is found on many cells in our bodies' upper respiratory tract and lungs. It also appears in the lining of our blood vessels, the heart itself, kidneys and our intestines. The blood becomes a river ride that stops at these ports that the virus takes to find a home in our living body. Know this truth, if we die so does the virus.

Now, I have seen some believe that the intestines may get affected by what we swallow. This is not generally accepted but I believe it to be true. I examine who is quick to learn and who knows how to find facts for my questions. I am logical I believe and so my point here is our experts must figure all routes to our organs. This includes liquids and food.

Healthy bodies stop this invasion by air in the nose or throat. Maybe the lungs too. This first line of defense is before the body itself realizes the body has been invaded.

Here those who do get sick suffer the flu like symptoms. They get a fever and a cough. Maybe even diarrhea. Then hopefully seven to ten days all is good again.

Others of us do not get better and suffer for longer. Here is where the body damage begins. People now will feel the shortage of breath. The ability to oxygenate the blood is damaged. The lungs are not getting the oxygen. This happened to me more than once when I played how high can I climb. When we get over a mile high we lose our ability to breathe the oxygen we are used to breathing at sea level until we get used to the new heights. Climbing too fast without taking the time to acclimate your body you could damage your lungs.

Now we at this stage have the symptoms of pneumonia. Pneumonia is really the general name for how lungs respond to an assortment of viral, bacterial and fungal infections. If you are curious like I am, this is good to know. Then ask your doctors which kind you have when you hear pneumonia is present.

Now we can learn how the lungs give and take the oxygen and carbon dioxide we and plants need to feed our systems. The duality of life.

With the C19 in our lungs the particles search for the blood to sail on through our bodies. The port of departure is the alveoli, (not a pasta). No, these alveoli are actually tiny sacs which hang like grapes do on a vine in our lungs. These sacs branch out into a network of bronchial tubes. These tubes are infested with ACE2.

What purpose did our body creator do this for? Well these sacs are where oxygen from the air breathed into our lungs passes into our blood system. And having a dual purpose these sacs are where the carbon dioxide is emptied out of our blood system so our lungs can breathe the carbon out into the air so the plants have something to breathe. The more damage done here the harder each breath becomes as the gases can not be exchanged in harmony. Understand that oxygen and CO2 are gasses. And our industrial lifestyles do poison these gasses which may have compromised our lungs to start with.

There is no absolute harmony in patients here. The disease does not attack each body the same way. As each body is individually tailored by our lifestyles. Again, back to my earlier thoughts, this proves my point that we need individual healthcare to assess the damaged patient's body so a remedy can be administered to each unique individual.

Depending on the health of our bodies, different factors come into play, including our brain being slowed down so our nervous system does not get the message that we are under attack. This is why it is so important for us to do every day some form of breathing exercises which helps clear up the passages in our nervous system that leads to our brain. Please become aware of your individual body. Listen to your body as it does communicate with you.

The truth is, today we are only beginning to understand what mankind has done in changing the environment that our bodies when our DNA was first created were made to live in. This is a new virus. It does not act the way we wish it would so we can remedy the damage with one simple shot unless we know at what stage the virus has taken up residency in our body. In the passages we need one remedy, in our blood, another remedy and in our organs we need a third remedy.

I am learning that when viruses connect to the ACE2 it makes the pneumonia different, as the damage may not be solely to the lungs but the narrowing of the blood vessels too. The new virus C19, "Dracula" can feed even more than before in earlier forms. How do we stop the feeding? Maybe dilating the blood vessels of patients will help. But that is for doctors to determine. Just be aware that this could work. Ask questions do not just sit and accept fate. You are in control.

So as if this is a football game the virus is on the offense. So our body is now in defense mode. The brain is the head coach so what defense play does our brain call out for our system?

The front line defenders are the immune system inside the cells so infected and they start producing the counter charge. What does this mean? Well, as things have changed from the calm way of ease that our bodies were made to live, a new plan to rebalance our system must be put in play. We are dis-eased, invaded in truth, so the stress signal goes out crying to wake up their hidden soldiers called Cytokines.

These defenders have a military exercise called Cytokinesis. What is this?

Cytokinesis is where the cell starts dividing. The cytoplasm of a single eukaryotic cell divides into two daughter cells. This creates more cells so the virus does not eat all the original DNA information stored inside our cells before the virus invasion. If the original information is not passed on to our new cells, our bodies will be out of balance and will lead to a premature ending of our physical lives.

This process also informs the neighboring cells that an attack is coming to it. So cells get your guard up. Or it says attack.

So now the ball is in the defenders' hands and these cells launch an all-purpose response. Part one is to start the cell process of inflammation. Part two is a targeted counter attack which uses our natural antibodies and cells specifically programmed in our DNA to attack both the virus invaders and the cells they so infected.

In essence this counteracts the infected cells by reproducing replacements called daughter cells. And this is the causes of our inflammation.

So for those of you like me who do not understand what is good about inflammation here is naked truth. Inflammation happens when chemicals from our body's white cells enter our blood or tissues to protect our body from the virus invaders. That simple.

Now this inflammation raises the blood flow to the damaged area. It causes redness and warmth. And swelling as the collateral result is caused by chemicals released into our system.

But severe inflammation of the lungs is not a good living thing for our bodies nor the hitchhiking virus. Severe inflammation causes acute respiratory distress aka ARDS. If this happens the patient is rushed to the intensive care unit aka ICU. Once there, ventilators are now needed to keep you breathing and getting the oxygen to your body parts.

Ventilators are not without problems. To get on one you are heavily sedated. Meaning it is dangerous as you can not feel and talk coherently if at all.

Downed out as I call this medical induced stage, you now must be watched. Again I repeat we need health care advocacy to take effect as people not machines because in this body state unintended things can go very wrong. Kidney failure can occur plus maybe blood clots and heart problems. Dehydration is another issue.

On the ventilators you are now in phase two of virus issues. Originally doctors at this stage here kept the patients here dry. Stopping liquids from entering the lungs. However they were not aware of the kidney damage or ignored it as the first thought was to keep the lungs moving the oxygen and carbon dioxide. We need liquid in our bodies. Absence of liquid can cause kidney issues. And kidney failure is one of the causes of death of today's C19 patients.

So what do we do? Punt or keep the scientific ball and look for more than before. This is what allows mankind to become great. We, as a team, go for the goal of winning. Keep investigating and get to the core of the Virus and what it does when it invades our body and how we get it out or kill it while inside without taking the patient with it.

Blood clots in some of our Covid 19 dead were found in the lungs. So now the doctors are using mild blood thinners as lung prophylactics. Blood clots happen here because on these machines there are no movements. Dehydration actually thickens the blood. Severe inflammation causes problems too. Because clotting substances in our cells walk hand and hand with the chemicals that bring on inflammation.

What causes heart issues as the patient starts rebounding from the lung issues in some patients is also not understood. Is this issue the result from the C19 or the inflammation that was triggered to kill the virus infected cells, are the answers to the questions that need to be determined.

Now scientists are focusing on why some get it and others, if they get it, get it in mild doses. Why are some of us predisposed to the virus as a life or death disease?

Lifestyle is the answer, my fellow soldiers looking for truth and hoping to discover justice. Lung problems or immune systems issues according to some are now not the biggest death factor. The biggest risk factors are hypertension, diabetes one if not checked and diabetes two and obesity which is really pre-diabetes two, plus heart disease.

Why? These four diseases are linked with ACE2. These diseases have more ACE2 on their cells as a response to the higher levels of inflammation that comes with their conditions. When C19 sticks to the ACE2, that tackle reduces the ability of ACE2 to do its job and protect the cells. The underlying inflammation gets worse. Also, those four diseases cause organ problems and as we learned the Covid 19 virus attacks the weakest organs.

When really out of order the body enters a cytokines storm. A storm so out of control the outcomes are horrible. This is when multi organ failure begins. So why not use the anti-inflammatory drugs? The issue is when. When do they get administered? If it's too late you're gone. If too early you may stop the immune system from doing its job.

Now we can read the news about those who survive their severe bout with C19. The belief is not a good forecast. You will have newer long-term health issues. Poor muscle strength and sub-par heart and lung function is the result. Lungs can recover as so can kidneys. But heart and muscle weakened by this disease? Not likely.

The brain too will feel the disease. The spinal cord and the nerves and the inflammation associated with the disease is where the muscles issues arise. Plus staying in the ICU for more than seven days can lead to cognitive impairment. Like a head injury in football. Delirium sets in and you can read about how the few who survived thought they were in a laboratory or space ship when they first can assimilate what the hospital helpers look like in their suit of protective contact armor.

I share this with you all now so we understand that we need to forget our previous imperial money first health system. Our lives are at stake. We need to share info. Applaud those who work to find the cures as well-as those who sacrifice their personal health and welfare helping us slay the dragon that our corrupt practice of polluting earth caused in the first place.

Let's wake up. Let's win and when we stem this tide let's fix our system so we stop killing nature in our endless pursuit of financial private pleasure.

A healthy earth ensures a healthy life. If you want to be happy for the rest of your life let's have a balanced earth.

Adults Children and Covid.

As we are now entering the fall in the northern hemisphere and in the Southern Hemisphere the summer of this year we call 2020 I feel it is important to share what our eyes can see as what is giving on with the COVID that is now acknowledged as living world-wide in our atmosphere.

How does it come down to the ground and when we are in close quarters who does it attack and why?

Close quarters are when we are locked up indoors because of the weather, be it too hot or too cold outside.

I was fascinated by the uptick in the states I call home here in the US. I live in both Florida and California and I work in Texas. All three states had a huge uptick this summer which made no sense if this disease was not airborne.

It is airborne and it is global. Know this truth. Our President Trump knew it and told the reporter Bob Woodward this truth right when the pandemic hit public awareness back in March of 2020. The crime here is both the President hid this truth and so did those who told the President this truth as well as the reporter who withheld this conversation so he could profit from the book he was writing.

And I see the disease as a heat seeking missile that comes down to earth and attacks those living forms it can penetrate their aura and get inside their body. The aura that is our body shield to keep viruses and other forms of energy from invading your body. Also it goes into our other foods that we eat, meaning foods above the surface. And it could hibernate inside our earth and come to us as part of the food we eat or the water we drink. Know this truth. Do not listen to the authorities who lie to us for a living. Be aware.

The breathing exercises I share with you in this book will protect you. But know this when you are down in body psyche, you become vulnerable. When you are depressed you become vulnerable. When you are in these down stages you must be aware of the condition your body is in and aware that this down stage will let negative thoughts and energy inside your body. This reduces your power, I call the energy of life. You need to fix your state of existence. You must relax and pump your system up with your breathing exercises. Even if for a minute or perhaps two. Pump your aura up.

Hard to do yes. But do it. Especially if you feel dark energy around you. Protect yourself. And this will protect others who you live with. This virus is Mother Earth telling us the polluting ways of your mankind industrial race has done enough damage. Clean up your mess. If not more will come from the Earth's body. We need to understand what the effect of polluting our water, air and land has done.

The Paris Climate treaty was a joke. All greedy representatives of nations negotiating time to continue to pollute earth, which includes our atmosphere, knowing full well that the day of reckoning was coming. That is why those who polluted the most were frantically searching for vaccines to stop the new disease we were producing earth to make as an effect of the cause of our pollution.

These treaties did not deal with truth. Yes we made a deal but with who? Us who pollute. We did not make a deal with our victim. That victim was Mother Earth. We need to understand that Father God will not help us fix Mother Earth except to speak to us and tell us this is nature's way of letting you know something is wrong.

So, for the future beings, and I am speaking of all beings not just mankind, we must stop our polluting ways. But for the present we must understand the way this energy called a virus comes down from the air and plays hide and seek as it tries to be the rat who wants our bodies' cheese. A cheese made by our digestive system and that lives in our organs which will feed the virus as the virus's new petri dish.

Know this truth. Weak organs are from our lifestyle of smoking and drinking alcohol or fake sugar sodas such as Coke or Pepsi and eating food fast foods and the candies which our lying FDA says is ok will kill you. The virus is making this truth happen sooner than we may like it. I must not leave out the candies every kid can buy in their public schools as snacks which put the young into a sugar high so they pay attention to their teachers regardless of the havoc this creates.

If you are old and have organ disease protect yourself. Exercise and keep your aura up. If it is down watch out. Also stay away from those who look and act like toxic human beings. Just go to the other side of the street. Be smart. This will end. But not when we say so. But when our air rebalances itself. That is until the next time which could be now.

The crowds are an energy of Earth's gravity. That energy brings the virus down to them from the air. I hate writing or saying this as I live off live audiences, but these crowds must be controlled. We need to not gather in crowds where the heat we generate brings the virus down to us from the atmosphere where it is living and hopefully being absorbed and to disappear in our atmosphere. It will sooner or later. But as it is not yet sooner we must be smart.

This is summer-time truth. Winter we need to not gather in large inside audiences where the virus does exist as we do not cleanse the indoor air and we must realize the virus is there. The less people we are with the better. The cold outdoor weather when you hibernate inside with others is a recipe too for you to get the virus if one of you have it.

During the fall and winter months it is imperative to get fresh air. In small crowds. The cold will keep the virus in the higher atmosphere which will come down only with the heat of the animals in an over crowded dense spot.

Subways and trains are a problem. Be aware. That's all I can offer up. Just be careful and if you get it that does not means it is over. You can strike back and protect yourself.

Trump's COVID fall is interesting. Trump swore it off. It will not hit him or his enlighten team, our King Midas preached. Join me and my gold attitude of invincibility will be an aura to protect you. Well today October 2nd we saw truth. Trump announced that he got COVID.

One week earlier on Saturday September 26, the Midas had his golden touch party on the lawn of the White House. Look liked a classic Viennese-style Catholic church concert with no mask. It was a warm late summer afternoon. The virus was circulating and it came down to play with those who attended the announcement of the Vatican's choice for our Supreme Court Justice vacant slot. The President picked Amy Coney Barrett as the winner of his choice to overturn the Roe v Wade decision that allows women to choose who can touch their bodies and a practice we call abortion.

Ms. Barrett had tested positive for Covid 19 the Seattle Times said earlier this year but has since recovered. The audience this introduction attracted was all red team without separation of church from state. We even had the head of the University called Notre (our) Dame (named for Mother Mary) John Jenkins at attendance. Jenkins has since come down with Covid19. I guess his version of Father God did not hear his plea. As did so far three US Republican Senators and the latest wife of Trump whom we call, the First Lady.

Why this hit Trump is easy to metaphysically analyze. Trump who has aura of invincibility was losing his shield. He was losing the popular polls that analyze this election for President which closed on November the 3rd. Trump was tired and was running scared. He does not like to lose, let alone admit defeat. His aura was down and the disease came into his body. His body was tired and now he got what he called the China Flu knowing full well as he spoke, he was lying to all including himself.

This is the story of King Midas. And now he will in his private moments, ask his version of Father God to help him. The invincible King will be humble and be human. It's what I thought. But boy, was I wrong.

So, you get Covid. Since the time I first wrote this book there are some remedies which they say will help shorten the invasion of this body snatchers called Covid 19.

Let's look at how the medics at Walter Reed Hospital with infusion of wisdom from the medics at Johns Hopkins Hospital were treating our President.

First off they were giving our President an experimental antiviral therapy called Remdesivir. What is this?

Remdesivir is an investigational nucleotide analog with broad spectrum antiviral activity. The use of this medicine, for lack of a better term, has finally been approved on December 11 by the FDA.

This remedy in tests has in vitro as well as in vivo activity in animal modes against the pathogens MERS and SARS which are also family members of coronavirus and are chemically similar structured to Covid-19. The preclinical data shows that this antiviral works on MERS and SARS to speed up the body's recovery from the invasion of those two so the bet is it will work the same on Covid-19.

What does all this mean? Well as a layman whose opinions are open for review I will now dissect what the authorities have shared.

What is an antiviral activity? Antiviral activity is how we measure the inhibitory effects of viral replication in cell cultures. This is usually used to evaluate in vitro pharmacologist activity of interferons.

What does inhibitory here mean? It means slowing down or preventing a process, reaction or function. So, it means stopping the duplication that the Covid-19 causes once inside your cells.

What is in vitro? Means taking place in a test tube, outside dish, or really anywhere not yet inside the living organisms. It is used to make babies of mankind. Something Trump's new Supreme Court Justice appointee wishes to prevent. Just saying.

What is in vivo? Means taking place inside the living organism.

What is it that anti-virals are really doing? Unlike antimicrobials, antivirals do not destroy or deactivate the microbe, which is in this case the virus. No, they act by trying to reduce and eventual sterilizing it from reproducing. Cutting off its balls so to say.

The goal is to prevent the viral load from increasing to a point where it can cause pathogenesis. Doing this it allows the bodies innate immune mechanisms to neutralize the virus.

Antivirals are plant based on the most part. So this method is a concoction of various herbs that Mother Nature produces or their chemicals Big Pharma create without the gift of life force to replicate a real Mother Earth remedy.

Common herbs are basil, sage and oregano, as well as lesser grocery store herbs but known to our mystical shamans such as Astragalus and Sambucus to name but two as there are many more. Understand this truth. Your chemicals have a proton and electron all with a neutron. Life has cells that have a proton and an electron, but the neutron is where the energy of life lives and perpetuates our living in this body form. Chemicals to date have not been given that energy we call life.

Nature has the cures to our disease. A dis-ease is really something that stops the flow of our well-balanced machine called a body. A body that our urbanization with industry first has abused as our scientists who work for the system lie and say this is all ok behavior.

Know there are answers to everything when you are willing to learn and if you have time to explore. No one can stop time. As our body does have a limited warranty in the first place. And this body of ours has a warranty different for each of us as it depends on our own DNA which was made to protect invasion of our bodies like viruses. We need to learn how to protect and honor the temple we live in by respecting

GOD and Mother Earth. And when I say GOD it is not the manmade versions of a father god.

One more naked truth to share with you. The coming virus vaccine. Watch out. Be smart and do what your body says not what society wishes you to do. There are no shortcuts. Know that. We have methods in place that test product all the time. But those tests are flawed. They measure short term relief. They are incapable of giving you a long term conclusion. As our bodies evolve they do not stay the same. We never measure the harm done in the future by using something right now. We are in a political battle to get a vaccine up and out to the public.

There will be issues galore. There will also be bootleg copies. Know this truth. The viruses will eventually on Earth's timeline not ours, be neutralized by our atmosphere. But know that does not mean another virus will not be released even as I write due to our polluting ways of living our lives in our urban greedy lifestyle.

Today, I am actually investigating Ivermectin. What is this you ask?

Ivermectin is an anti parasite drug treatment that seems to work for Covid. The drug apparently helps stop the spread of Covid as it is inhibits the reproduction of SARS COV-2 in vitro.

And knowing this naked truth, Earth, as I said must be involved in all our time delay negotiations. We need to clean up our mess now. Mother Earth is changing and we make it happen. Deal with it.

Now to the children. Covid-19 in Babies and Kids: Symptoms and Prevention.

Doctors say that as more details emerge about this virus parents can feel better that in the majority of the cases, the disease "seems" to be much milder in babies and children. Reassuring message. Right? No.

Why does it attack any bodies? And why are some children not part of the majority? This child could be yours or someone in your family, or your friend's baby.

So let's critically look and see what goes on with the newer bodies not yet worn and torn by our way of living in this pollution age of Urbanization of Earth. The newest terror TV show that hopefully soon will be cancelled.

What are the Covid-19 symptoms? This applies to babies as well as nursing home survivors. And in fact, everyone. This is all ages.

Symptoms are the following:

1. Cough

2. Fever or chills

3. Shortness of breath as well as difficulty in breathing.

4. Muscle or body aches

5. Sore throat

6. A sudden loss of taste or smell.

7. Diarrhea.

8. Headaches

9. New fatigue

10. Nausea or vomiting

11. Congestion or running nose.

This is the check list. Use your judgement as you diagnose yourself and children or parent as well as significant other.

But children are known to have pneumonia, with or without obvious symptoms. They can also experience sore throats, excessive fatigue as well as diarrhea. I for one got my tonsils out to stop sore throats when I was a child. I don't know if that was a good thing or bad but we did it back then. A 50's child I am.

Data from the CDC study indicate as well as they indicate for those no longer a child that there is higher risk for children depending on their circumstances. Those at higher risk are the following:

1. Children under two. Why? Because their system is not yet a perfected running machine. We age differently. Some are slower than others. And we do not yet know if their machine/body is perfect.

2. Black and Latino Children, who can be affected by "health disparities". These health disparities leave them dispro-portionally vulnerable to Covid-19 complications. I will go over the health disparities below.

3. Children who were born prematurely. Why? Their system may be compromised from the start.

4. Those who are fat from eating which we call obesity to be politically correct.

If you feel your kid is sick for no reason deal with it. Go to a doctor. Unfortunately our for-profit nation does not have universal health care for all so you may be afraid to go to a doctor because you have no health care which our idiot nation calls insurance. My advice is improvise and go where you can get help. Even if it's to an emergency ward. Again, I really can not believe our nation called the U.S. has no Universal Health Care for all. Maybe that is why we are the United States of Covid.

Some signs to act regardless of insurance are the following:

1. Difficulty breathing and trying to catch your breath.

2. Inability to keep liquids down.

3. Confused state or inability to get up and about.

4. Bluish lips as well as face. As well as unusual body or muscle aches

5. Children with medical conditions such as Asthma or Diabetes much be really watched.

Can kids spread the Covid-19. Yep they can. How? Same as you and me. The data to date shows that while the kids have a milder form of the virus they carry as much of this virus in their mouths and nose as adults do. Deal with this truth.

How to keep COVID-19 away from kids? Same way as you keep it from you?

Let's review what we are being told to do in the ideal world the docs wish us to live in. Meaning do what you can when you can. Do not obsess if you are doing something and cannot follow protocol. Just be smart. And stay aware. Do not let anxiety enter your psyche. If you do you have opened the hole into your protective shield called your aura.

The current list of what we are told to follow:

1. Distancing. Must be maintained. And before you send your kids to school or play groups or day care see what they are doing to protect social distancing. Remember when it was only the contagious flu your child was the probable source of your catching it. Your child is being put into a social experience of other children whose parents may not think or act as you do. Your child is exposed to the children's parents living order.

2. Wear the mask. Important.

3. Wash hands and keep clean.

4. Do not play with faces.

My advice is be wise. Be careful stay healthy. Watch what you eat. Take care of yourself.

And before I leave you with my best wishes and prayers for your continued survival I must now share an ugly truth. That truth is "health disparities".

What is health disparities? And how does it affect and effect us living in the US of A?

As our schools of knowledge be it Johns Hopkins or any looking for data to give finite conclusions, they are discovering trends that shows a disproportionate number of people contracting and dying from Covid-19 among what they call minorities communities. Really meaning the poor, which is really the caste system of American me, me, me capitalist society. A society where we do not take care of each other as we believe they must do it for themselves. They need to get a job no matter how bad the conditions for work are and the fact that they are underpaid does not matter.

Our imperial religion and government says god wants it this way. Well maybe it is time to fire that god and become a society where we provide everyone a standard of decent living if you are part of the society working to build a society for all not just to perpetuate one for the few.

This is truth. We need a new system. We need it now. We need to wake up and see we are the cause of all our disease.

Time to speak up. Time for change. Time to take back our lives.

Let's look at recent developments this past fall of 2020.

As we are now entering the fall in the Northern Hemisphere and in the Southern Hemisphere the summer of this year we call 2020 I feel it is important to share what our eyes can see as what is going on with the COVID that is now world-wide in our atmosphere.

How does it come down to the ground and when we are in close quarters who does it attack and why?

I was fascinated by the uptick in the states I call home here in the US this past summer. I live in both Florida and California and I work in Texas. All three states had a huge uptick this summer which made no sense if this disease was not airborne.

It is airborne and it is global. Know this truth. Our president knew it and told the reporter Bob Woodward this truth right when the pandemic hit public awareness back in March of 2020. It was actually before, as I believe I got it coming back from London October 2, 2019. The crimes here are the US President Trump hiding this truth and the people who told the President this truth as well as the reporter who withheld his conversation with Trump so he could personally profit from the book he was writing. I do believe this is moral criminality.

And I see the disease as a heat seeking missile that comes down to land or our seas from our atmosphere and attacks those living forms it can penetrate their aura and get inside their body.

The aura is our body shield to keep viruses and other forms of energy from invading your body. Also it goes into our foods that we eat meaning foods above the surface. And it could hibernate inside our earth and come to us as part of the food we grow to eat or the water we drink. Know this truth. Do not listen to the authorities who lie to us for a living. Be aware.

The breathing exercises I share with you in this book will protect you. But know this when you are down in body psyche, you become vulnerable. When you are depressed you become vulnerable. When you are in these down stages you must be aware of the condition your body is in and aware that this down stage will let negative thoughts and energy inside your body. You need to fix your state of existence. You must relax and pump your system up with your breathing exercises. Even if for a minute or perhaps two. Pump your aura up.

Hard to do? No, unless you are lazy. So my advice is just do it. Especially if you feel dark energy around you. Protect yourself. And this will protect others who you live with. This virus is Mother Earth telling us the polluting ways of your mankind industrial race has done enough damage. Clean up your mess. If not more will come from my Earth body. We need to understand that the effect will are living in of polluting our water, air and land is done.

As I alluded to before, Trump's Covid 19 so called infection is interesting. Trump as our fearless leader swore it off. He claimed it was not real. It was just an inconvenient truth that he our leader swore off for anyone that followed his reckless leadership of absolute denial. It will not hit him or his enlightened team, our Nero, with his tongue as his violin preached. Join me as he played King Midas with his gold attitude of invincibility and denial. If you believe what I say, this Trump truth will be a golden aura to protect you. Well we all can see the naked truth if we stop drinking his Kool Aid.

Why this Covid 19 invaded Trump is easy to metaphysically analyze. Trump who has his self proclaimed aura of invincibility was losing his shield. He was losing the popular polls that analyze this election for President which closed on November 3rd. Trump was tired and was running afraid. He does not like to lose, let alone admit defeat. His aura was down and in the disease came. His body was tired and now he got what he called the China Flu knowing full well as he spoke, he was lying to all including himself.

This is really a remake of the myth, the story of King Midas. And now he will in his private moments ask his version of Father God to help him. The invincible king could not be humble and be human. No this "pig" in reality did all. He could downplay the effects of this Covid 19 disease and in turn made a mockery of all those who suffered because of Covid and our US inability to have the supplies to help our healthcare systems ready and able to confront the disease that our industrialization of earth made happen. Trump is not in control of his final destiny nor destination.

And this lack of empathy, this lack of compassion and the Nation's overdose of Trump media got the Nation to vote this demigod out.

In our future watch what this ego driven man of one does to our country as he sits and runs his Shadow Government to keep him on our TV news shows. Watch the gutless republicans not stand up to this clown and in effect we become the saddest side show in our world where once we claimed we were the home of democracy. What a lesson he will become in the future's history books. Never let a merchant with no morals or class let alone empathy for the people run your government.

Let's move to Part Three after this book picture break.

Highways and byways
How SARS-CoV-2 affects the body

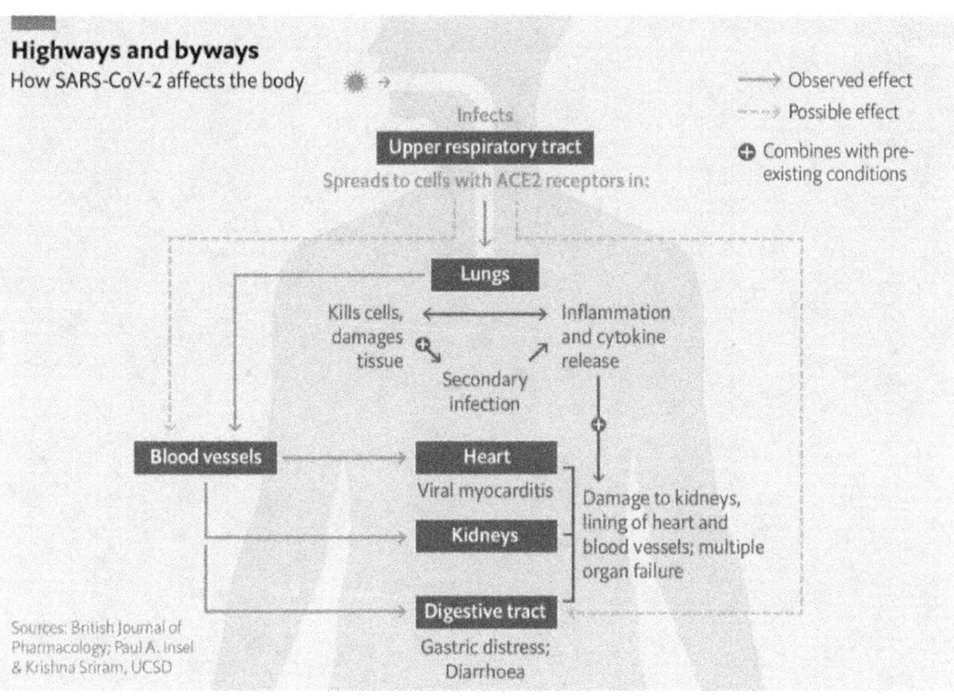

Part Three

Metaphysical Truths and Manmade Lies.

As I just said at the end of Part One these following two paragraphs must be understood:

My educated and researched personal opinion is this viral C19 disease is manmade. It comes from our sick and demented lifestyle where we believe we can chemically change the gases which causes a new balance of our air and water and land both above and below. All done I must add so we can perpetuate the urban industrial and military world order that is the cause of each new earth disease.

We argue amongst ourselves about climate change and even there our agreed solution is to act right many years into the future. We need to wake up. We need to recognize our industrial behavior does change the balance of earth each day. And that change does not have a replay. We cannot go back.

We in the United States need a national healthcare system without insurance from private third for profit parties. A national healthcare system, one that plans ahead. The monies are paid for out of the money supply our nation prints and gives to the fed to loan back to us. This is really the best gangster game ever. I have spent twelve years of my life trying to educate our nation.

We need to plan ahead as a living community band invest in the products we need to ensure that our local communities can deal with this latest disease as we strive for herd immunity until we have the nerve to stop the poisons we put into the earth in the first place. The virus too wishes to survive. Know that's truth. Sorry, some will die including I, but the game of life includes inevitable death and the government's job is to help postpone death by sharing information amongst the people so we can do more and survive to thrive.

We need to become really responsible. And being responsible means firing the people in government who can not get along. Maybe the end game we have in this nation, winner by election takes all, must end too. Life is a balance and red vs blue, which I must add, were the colors of the War of U.S. Independence, must end. Red and blue in our bodies (blood is red and blue is the clean air that we're supposed to breathe) represents the living and the dead

Also please accept this truth, our US country was created to run a central government of 13 states with 2.5 million people. Then those people had different lifestyles. We need to break up our central government into geographic centers. Just like we do with our sports leagues. I wrote about this in my book Man, Community and Living the American Dream.

Also, we must understand that the social governments of Europe with their health care systems and safety nets for the people were created or perpetuated by our Marshall Plan to rebuild Europe after WWII. This form of government helping the nation wide community of people which our Trump Kool Aid drinkers as well as the Corporate Democrats say this is socialism or the onset of communism. Forget these idiotic labels as it is proper 21St century government.

And my prayers which I now share with you are the following I want you to hear.

The world needs to unite. Our scientists be they a noun or a verb, need to disrobe themselves of business before people and their religion before other religions and treat each of us as equals. The common element of all religions and governments is we accept there is a God. To ensure health the world must operate as one in touching honoring both Father God and Mother Earth.

The vaccine for C19, now that it is ready, will either be a live or dead vaccine. What's the difference? The live vaccines are those that respond when the disease enters the body as a toxin, bacteria or virus. They don't last for a lifetime because these vaccines are weaker than the live attenuated (less virulent) vaccines.

A dead vaccine is made up of pathogens that are inactivated or killed before they go into battle. The slayings occur in a variety of ways. Those ways include heat, radiation, or chemicals. Unlike the staying power of live attenuated vaccines reinforcement may be required for these dead vaccines by booster shots.

Both live and dead vaccines respond when the disease enters the body be the disease a toxin, bacteria or virus. Our scientific scholars worldwide tell us that vaccines provide immunity against targeted diseases through antibodies that have been produced or stimulated by the vaccine itself. The antibodies are created from the agent that caused the disease you are attempting to neutralize or protect against possibly a synthetic version. Vaccines are not necessarily curative medicines that heal an existing condition. They are preventive. They protect you from contracting the disease and most times work as antigens.

Vaccines create a form of herd immunity and stop the spreading of the disease from one to another as the other already has the new virus.

This is what I believe. Those who do not agree, are really those who live in the thought system that says all that exists is what I can see, hear, taste, touch or feel. Well you cannot see, hear, taste or touch a virus before it enters you. But once inside you will feel it.

Again, I must state my worldly elder statesmen conclusion is all life began and continues to begin as a virus. This C19 virus is alive and without placing blame we must create the serum that will give us the herd immunity we need to survive.

Now maybe we can understand why our imperial government and the polluters running their polluting business invested their energies for private profits in learning about viruses our urban industrial behavior was creating instead of stopping it. We are being led on purpose to believe this coronavirus disease just magically came out of nowhere and now is looking for a place to be part of the physical world we all live in.

The few who run our world are well aware that the industries we live off for paper currency pollute earth. That pollution creates the black hole of life for new viruses to appear. An entry port of sorts. Knowing they are doing wrong they also spend time to figure out what new virus may come out of the harm they are doing to earth.

That my friends are truths. One day our survivors, the heirs, will all be educated to understand the real building blocks of life so we all can protect our bodies. The real Earth temple of the partnership of Father God our collective consciousness and our individual souls, with Mother Earth the owner of our body parts.

But do understand when we change the eco-balance of earth for an Imperial order to thrive and control earth, history will teach us that a virus will appear. This virus which will alter which Earth others in control believed to be the only version of Earth.

Remember Earth is a large living and evolving consciousness. We are in Earth's playground. We play by her rules not the ones we want Earth to play by. If we wish Earth to provide then we must understand we must provide to Earth too. That is how physical life works. We give and we get. If you give and do not get you will fall on your face. If you take and do not give you will fall on your back. This is the see-saw of life. The true scales of physical and spiritual justice. The supreme astrological sign of all living beings. The Libra. The balancer of the life force energy, the energy which makes our wants and needs.

I will now share some metaphysical truths. Viruses are no accident. Mother Earth creates them due to our altering physical behavior of the earth balanced machines. The machines that are roaming and breathing the air this planet creates with its water, air and land as well as the gravitational force that keeps our consciousness here in all our earth body forms.

And know I must add the following truths for you to really understand. We must be Pro-Life and I am not talking abortions I am talking earths lives.

Protect our Earth. Be aware that half of Earth's species have disappeared in the last forty years of our urbanization of Earth with chemicals. Those chemicals changed the womb of Earth and those changes are what make different life forms, including viruses.

New species are also being created. These urbanized life-style using chemicals cause climate change quicker then nature wanted it to occur. Know earth does have climate change by definition of its spinning and rotating ride in the Universe attracting and receiving energies from the beyond not just our atmosphere and solar system.

Part Four

A guide to help you as individuals to maximize your physical living health.

So now what can we do as individuals to protect ourselves from diseases entering our body?

A lot is my answer. But it does require self-work. You must keep up to be up. You must stay healthy in your body and your mind as well as your communicating with thy higher self. The source of all our earth physical energy.

We must eat, as much as we can, food made by earth, not food grown from man-made seeds or out of man-made chemicals.

We must drink pure water that contains the energy of life. Not water carrying the blood of excess death or poison from the chemicals created to help man in their industrial complex ways. The air must be pure of dinosaur oils and new urbanized gases as Mother Earth chose to bury just as Zeus buried the Titans, his parent's generation of his world order.

This is hard to do but we must collectively stop what we are doing so earth can cleanse. Solar and air energy is the key to a proper life style without gases made from chemicals we create.

Till then we must learn the way to raise our levels of energy inside our body as well as create a protective shield around our body. A shield that does help stop the invasions of viruses

Here are some of my simple yet practical ideas in hope we can each do just that in all times of our lives not just when a pandemic appears because as a new one can come at any time.

The Individual:

Let's realize that our body is our soul's engine from our higher consciousness we take to explore physical life on a planet we call Earth.

So first let's explore what a planet really is all about.

NASA, which stands for the National Aeronautics and Space Administration and is a US Federal Agency gives us a good definition of the meaning of a planet which I will now share with you.

Their definition says a planet is a celestial body that is in orbit around an energy force called a star which here on Earth we call our Sun. The planet has a sufficient mass for itself with a gravity to overcome rigid body forces so that it assumes a hydrostatic equilibrium, (meaning nearly round) shape. Plus, the energy the planet creates living and orbiting the sun has cleared its neighborhood around its orbit unless a supernatural energy appears from elsewhere and it does happen. Know this truth.

Now follow me. A planet is a collective energy that has used its gases and liquids to create solids and then balance all three so that the planet can wander space in an orbit around its energy source. The planet has created gravity to bring what it needs around its body as a shield to protect itself from substances for the most part from entering its atmosphere shield. That is unless the invasion mass has the speed and energy to invade and break on through the to the other side of that shield.

Somehow, we must all see and hopefully begin to understand these universal metaphysical truths.

Now if I may, let's say we are really just a human planet. An individual planet that came together from gas called consciousness. We figured out how to enter this planet called earth by being a gas, a virus of thought that has discovered a way to get our thought intellectual soils inside a body that exists on earth so we can do what?

So we can discover life in physical form. Our consciousness has created our life out of nothing. We live inside a galaxy called consciousness and we invaded earth to have this living experience. We are a collective group that has created a herd immunity invading earth.

But we need to keep our engine, our body, alive as long as we can. We must keep it tuned. A maintenance of sorts so it runs efficiently. We must learn how to ignite our bodies with energy so the shield works outside called an aura. We need to tune up our engines daily so the inside works. And there are times because of elements around us both seen and not visible to the eyes that cause our body to go off and this requires a cleansing of our organs that are polluted because of fears as well as viruses that somehow got into our system.

A fear is really a thought virus set inside our minds to stop our bodies working with ease. Fear is disease. We need to keep fears outside our body. Fear enters our minds and do damage our system. An aura shield will help stop the fear from entering most times.

A physical virus finds the opening in our bodies which is by breath or digestion. The fear virus enters our mind by thought. This virus now in physical form will attach itself to the building block of our machine called a cell. Once inside the cell the virus will take command of the machine that reproduces our cells and gives the cells the energy to run efficiently without fears. We have just learned all how this works.

So how do we stop viruses of both thoughts and physical substance from entering our individual bodies? We keep our individual body working the best we can both inside the physical body as well as outside the body to prevent viruses from entering our individual atmosphere which we call aura. The aura is our body's protection shield. It is so important that we realize this truth.

Our leaders somehow have the energy to give you the awareness that they are a source of energy. That energy force attracts you to the leader. Unfortunately, that is not our politicians. They are used by other energized leaders not in public view to go around and keep this system of matrix control alive where the few get you to serve them believing Father God will take care of you next time.

These politicians which include the religious priests of all imperial religions get you to believe in what serves the few as opposed to serving all of us. This is why sacred knowledge becomes secret. This is why when you don't agree with the politically correct wisdom of the moment you are labeled crazy or too spiritual for mass mankind consumption.

The strongest power man can have is to have the power to tell what that man believes to be universal truths and not care what the mass puppet masters say and make the public believe. Mankind survived for eons without the industrial agricultural world and Big Pharma the cause of our latest disease.

Some wish to lead for self-grandeur such as Donald J. Trump. Others wish to teach to lead all for some common goal which is just for one. I wish to teach so we learn Universal truths on how we can stay on earth to survive the game of life in both physical and group form. Plus, I want to share ways for us to strive and thrive as individuals so we can all win the yearly game of life with its four seasons of birth, growth and harvest and hibernation where we get the energy to do it again.

Some rules to share before I explain the exercises we must do. And I know it is hard so do the best you can each and every moment you feel the attack coming. Remember you have one asset. Our asset is God. The love of our creator which gives us the energy of our body source called the heart. Keep your heart open. Do not let fear shut it.

Rule one: Believe in yourself.

Rule two: Fight off fears.

Rule three: And it is hard to do, get rid of others with toxic energy. They are vampires. They are viruses coming to steal your energy. They will break your protective shield.

Rule four: Watch what you eat and drink. Be aware.

Rule five: Help your fellow man but do not let that help break your shield. Be strong and when you notice the hole in your shield get strength from your heart so you can carry on like a good soldier of life.

Now let's move to the exercise. Exercises designed by the ancients before imperial religions and imperial governments came forth to shut down awareness. These ancient practices are to help keep your body and mind sound and your heart open. All so you can enjoy the physical and metaphysical aspects of daily life.

We must train our brains to focus now. Hard to do. Many use meditation to do this. I do too. But in exercise we must keep the mind focused to clear thoughts so we can mend a body to fully perform its task for efficient performance day in and day out.

Focus on your breath. Breath is what you need in your body to keep it working at its peak capabilities which does change over time.   Breathe in through your nose and then breathe out through your nose when fear enters inside your body. Get rid of it.

Pump the air in and let it out to get the wrong thoughts out of your system.

Look at a baby and watch it breathe. A baby breathes in and out through its nose and pumps its stomach as it breathes. A baby has no fear.

Through the eyes of a child everything is beautiful. That is until we adults instill our fears inside that baby's mind.

We, as we age, breathe only through our mouths when we get upset or allow fears to take hold of our body. Relax when you feel this happening. Hard to do yes. But do it. Then close your eyes. Count a number of breaths to erase fears, long deep breaths in and out through your nose and then open your eyes. The thoughts that caused fears are gone.

I am a student of *Kundalini*. A practice that I believe our creators gave their servants eons ago in the area we call India today. The energy we call *Inanna* or *Isis* I believe is the one that taught these breath practices to us. It is sacred knowledge.

Knowledge that the masses were prohibited from understanding and living. Why? You will see through the shadow of the puppet masters smile. And yes, we have puppet masters. Or why would any of us believe someone is better than we are as individuals. These few actually believe they deserve more than you so you will work and slave to the rhythms of a fixed system and hope that maybe you can find the hole and enter their elevated atmosphere.

Now let's follow my thoughts. Our body is the temple of Father God and our Mother Earth the two being our parents we hear about in the Ten Commandments of Enlil, the god who tried to civilize man back during Moses time here on earth.

Good health is the gift from our two parents, Father God and Mother Earth. Our parents talk to us and let us know when our system is in need of awareness that something is wrong. Remember Man is nothing but the being of our co-creators.

We are taught that our bodies have ten soul parts. What are those parts? Here we go on our metaphysical journey to truth the enlightened way.

First is the soul body.
Two is the negative mind.
Three is the positive mind.
Four is the neutral mind.
Five is the physical body.
Six is the arc line.
Seven is the auric body.
Eight is the organic body.
Nine is the subtle body.

Ten is the radiant body.

Let's go over all ten bodies in this metaphysical discussion of taking care of your personal business. Your personal earth life.

What is a Soul Body? A body is your physical structure. It is made of flesh, bones and blood. As well as water and filled with air. Your soul is your individual spiritual consciousness living inside your body, responding to your body's awareness.

A consciousness I must now add is bigger than your soul. It is the real you. The consciousness is both your inside soul and the consciousness that you are part of that really watches over you. It is your higher power. These exercises to tune up your body and keep the body up will help open the passage to the eternal everlasting you.

What is Negative Mind? Well it is when your mind which when you close your heart and the mind takes over your body and gets you to live as a beast. You are in protection mode. You tend to find the worst in everything. You hear words and interpret those vocal vibrational thoughts by seeing or feeling the worst possible scenarios that can happen to you.

What is a Positive Mind? This is a mind who leads by the heart. You see the beauty in all. You approach situations with a positive attitude. You need to be aware that the mean wolf may be near and do not let that energy consume you. Use that as protection not exclusion. Your attitude changes the way most people and other animals and plants as well as water feel your entry into their personal aura. A collision of worlds which is really chaos. Chaos being two or more energies sharing the same aura space.

What is a Neutral Mind? It is a mindset that is not sexy nor exciting. The mind is calm. The mind is precise. The neutral mind is our sacred weapon for sustainability and steadiness in a world of constant changes and resulting chaos. The invasion of auras.

What is a Physical Body in this metaphysical world? A physical body is a collection of matter within a defined contiguous boundary in three- dimensional space. The boundary is defined by the parts of the final product. Your inner space which works together as one living machine.

But understand this one machine is made of separate parts. An army that must march through life together as a team. A team working so the body will win for as long as possible. All bodies in 3D form are built with a limited warranty.

What is Arc Line? In the tradition of the Kundalini practice of the sages an arc line is seen as a halo. One that stretches around your forehead, earlobe to earlobe. The yogis of this Kundalini practice teach that women have an extra arc line that runs from Nipple to Nipple. Why? To assist in the bonding of a child and the baby's mother.

An Arc Line in physical science is defined as segments of rays. Rays that may or may not be bound together. A common curved example of an arc line is the arc of a circle. A quick review of geometry we were taught, if you paid attention, that the arc of a circle is called a circular arc. In a sphere an arc is called a great circle. In an ellipse it is called a great arc. Please do note, every pair of two distinct points, which includes two humans near each other, have two colliding arcs. The more people inside the new circle gives you more colliding points called chaos.

We learn how to live within chaos by creating acceptance to the collision of people's arc lines. We accept that collision. We navigate it or leave it.

As a side note, when you hear words Mercury Retrograde or Venus Retrograde it means that the planet is now colliding with our earth's arc line. Retrograde makes you backpedal before you go forward again.

What is the Auric Body? This is metaphysical term and naked truth, but it is so important for your overall health to understand. Our human bodies are composed of biological circuits. Circuits that carry electric currents throughout the complex wiring of our body's systems, which includes our nervous system. This electricity creates the electronic field around our body which is our personal atmosphere and is known as aura.

All matter has this electric field. Some denser than others. Even rocks have this field. And we are attracted to the energies of rocks. You wear stones for this reason. Diamonds are crystals. They radiate energy. Gold radiates energy. But know these crystals and metals do take your full tank of energy away. You are a rock and you are a floating island. Watch out for the jewelry you may wear. It steals energy from your energy force. Saying this so you are aware of truths.

The Auric Body contains the Prana Body. What is the Prana Body?

The Prana Body is the one that brings the life force and its energy into your system through breath. Be it your nose or your mouth. This breath when mastered will bring fearlessness, purity, energy to combat invasion of your inner self as well as self-initiation.

What is Subtle Body?

A metaphysical definition is that this describes one of the three bodies that collectively constitute a human existence. This is the astral body. The other two bodies are the physical body and the causal body.

The Subtle Body is a combination of the mind, the intellect and your individual ego. This subtle body controls the physical. And through this body you experience pain and pleasure. The subtle body is all temporary states that are only associated with physical existence. There is no pain or pleasure outside your body. If you could ever reach this state you are on your way back to Nirvana. The eternal state of evermore you and God are now together with no wants and no needs. You went home. Mother Earth and you are no longer together.

The Causal Body, I now will add, is the one that becomes the veil over your higher consciousness. Man, as a soul only is a causal body being. We inside this body mindset are really the matrix for the astral and physical bodies. Open up this part of your existence and you will see the greater matrix of energy existence. Not just the world and that system you were born to breathe and believe is the only system that exists.

What is a Radiant Body?

According to my guru teachers, a radiant body refers to a field of energy that extends (circle) nine feet around our body. The energy comes in thru our crown chakra, that is why kings and queens wear open crowns. That is also why when you pray to a fake god you are required to wear a closed cap so you do not get all the information from the higher powers that surround you. That's the game my friends. You are prevented from realizing by higher spirits that you are praying to a fake god. If God wanted you to wear a hat he would have made you with that hat.

A radiant body gives you courage and strength. You project this energy with everything that touches you. You have the shield to stop invasion of fears and vampire energy. And do know our world is run by vampire energy that uses our lives to feed their wants and needs telling us and us believing that this is what the imperial god, not GOD wants us to do. We are being manipulated by sights we are programmed to see one way, as well as noise that we are programmed to hear to feel certain feelings.

Metaphysical Truths continued.

There are two ways to live your life. One you go and get what you want. Here you are playing a bumper car game. Need to have the energy to last all the collisions your wants and needs will attract. I played this game. I succeeded and hated each breath I took. All to out-smart you so I could have.

However, my higher consciousness always taught me to share what I obtain and that struggle makes me who I am today. Fame and fortune in the imperial system based on scarcity is not what it is made out to be. It is a vampire lifestyle of never having enough. In reality you have more than you'll ever need. You lose yourself trying to obtain physical happiness while losing your eternal self.

The real game of life is to evolve your radiant body so things will come to you. This I always knew but was never able to fully understand until I was ready. This radiant body field is why I, apparently upon reflection as I write this now, attract creative forces as well as dark energies. I am still learning to navigate my ways through both sides of the tracks.

The trick I see is to dedicate yourself to higher consciousness. Hard to do. But try to live it. And if you see yourself falling backward look hard at the other energy around you. Get away from negative energy.

Time to analyze Inner Anger. The anger that destroys our balance. What is Inner Anger?

Inner Anger is the base of both inferiority as well as superiority complexes. Inner Anger is the core of manipulation with bad intent. It is where lies are born. It is the cause of most inner diseases that manifest on our skins. Inner Anger makes us not see the forest through your tree.

If I may digress for a moment, here in the US we believe in either red or blue. Manipulated by this exclusion, and not seeing that this political divide is based on anger. Resulting in us not sharing but being controlled by our puppet masters who control our purse strings. This is control that we gave those few by agreeing to be bound inside the matrix of our minds that we are taught to believe and accept.

Do you really believe in an Imperial God and that God's chosen governments who say kill for me? If God wants them dead tell God to do it. Let get rid of this Inner Anger.

How? Best way to do it is exercise. Get your body up and going. Movement will release you from this inner anger. Talk to the divine and stop letting other parts of this present system based on fears and it's resulting hate control you. God is love and love is God. Go to God. Not a Priest or Rabbi or Inman or any third party to communicate with Father God for you. Go directly to the source. Talk to Father God and let it flow.

And learn to talk to Mother Earth and all of her other Children. Learn to talk to the Wind, as the Wind is your Friend.

It's important for all to understand the concept of Karma. Karma is when you can't let go of your negative energy caused by your behavior. If someone is bad to you, move on and let it go. By keeping it alive inside you create the negative energy that will grow and fester inside your nervous system, not just your minds.

It will place a hole in your metaphysical heart. If you don't let go, that negative energy called Karma will come back to get you in the end. And know that we are in this ocean of thought, if someone is doing something wrong to you it is imperative to say something immediately and make them aware that their behavior is wrong.

Most of us live in a subjective world. We see only ourselves as a villain or hero. It is our duty as citizens to share with someone that has pierced our aura with negative energy that they believe is positive to let them know our true feelings. Then at that point get out of that situation. Move on.

You did not need lifetimes living your karma which was a reaction to what you did to someone. If you realize that you did someone wrong and that thought is burning inside you no matter how hard it is for you to do, you must contact that person and cleanse your Karma in this lifetime. Why wait?

So in conclusion, to release bad Karma, just let it go. How? Just learn through physical and mental exercises now how to let it go. Forgive yourself and make the changes so you do not do it again.

I must now share with you all what a high priest of the Orthodox Eastern Christian Church told me about Mother Mary. We got into a discussion and I asked him how he could perpetuate a lie and tell people Mary, the mother of Jesus, was a virgin. He stumbled. He did not know what to do. I pushed. I pushed. Please share with me what I then said metaphysical game this physical expression of being Mary being a virgin is all about.

Finally, this high ranking imperial priest said to me with tears in his eyes the following: Being a virgin like Mary means you came to earth without anyone's Karma attached to you. You are pure, you are a virgin at that moment as you have no Karma.

Ok I said, I get it. However naked truth, when we are born, we acquire the Karma of our parents and their biological families and friends. Then we acquire the Karma of those who enter in our lives. We obtain their fears and joys but are never taught how to let those fears go and stay outside our aura. We need to learn to accept the lessons and remember the good times not just the bad. This truth happens to all of us.

We need to create a school of higher learning. I am trying my part to do this with the creation of the 21st century return of Schools of Sacred Knowledge. Schools that are dedicated to the profit of mankind. Not some corporate game where we say this is a tax device. No, my game is to make you aware that you can breathe in and see truths when you keep fear outside your aura and expelled by a breath of fire from your inner workings.

We need to get in touch with our body and its mind. We need to control our bodies' responses from the heart, not a knee jerk reaction of our minds. When you do this, you can inherit your destiny you came to earth to fulfill.

Until you do you are living your fate. This is the difference between destiny, which is really the reason why we came here, not fate, which is what the imperial system, really a closed off matrix disconnected from the universe, bestowed on us by telling us we must follow their rules.

You are allowing some other energy to tell you how to live your life. You will be back to try it again. Lose that Karma. It's hard to do. So very hard to do. I get it. I am still in that process. I am hu-man. But I see the other realities too.

Again I must emphasis, please be aware that we need to exercise our body to get the blood flowing to feed our organs. Please understand that each organ is a separate being all part of your body's universe.

There are exercises for each organ as part of the curriculum of Kundalini. I promise the time spent with your intention to heal will cleanse you to live a better more fulfilled life.

At the end of this book I share with you two groupings of Kundalini exercises that I was taught to help tune your body and keep it up so you can be up. There are many more.

I ask you to take the time if you are curious to please look up Kundalini.

Saying that, please be aware I do and have done a lot more exercises than just Kundalini. Both Yoga and all physical sports that I could participate in at various stages of my life.

Experiment and explore all the possibilities with a Guru or a sport as well as life coach who understands the sacred knowledge of the exercise you are about to undertake.

Now let's focus on more than heart rate.

There are exercises to tune up your glandular system. What is your glandular system?

This is the system that is also called the endocrine system. It pertains to your pituitary gland and your thyroid glands, you parathyroid glands and your adrenal gland, your pancreas, as well as your sex glands be they ovaries for you with a womb or your testicles if you are just a mere man.

These glands produce hormones that regulate the metabolism of our bodies. They regulate the growth and development of our bodies. These hormones so produced by our glands regulate our tissue function, sexual function as well as our sleep too. They regulate our moods. This is so important to keep well and functioning in balance.

A truth I have discovered. I understand the ins and outs on a daily basis being a Type One Diabetic and wanting to live my life my way not some fearful way or in denial.

I set out to learn the truth of how and why the body works the way it does. My body caused by a virus shut off my ability to produce insulin. But the rest of my system works if I give myself the insulin my body no longer produces.

Due to this virus which shut down my capabilities in my DNA of producing insulin I must be constantly aware of the state of my organs. I am doing the best I can so I can fulfill my destiny. Not fall victim to someone else's destiny by living their fears and denying my full potential of life.

Now lets move into the metaphysical sacred knowledge of Breaths:

The air we breathe is how we become more than we are. Breath is Prana, when breath is considered as a life-giving force.

There are *Prana Vayu* exercises that specifies target breathes. "Vayu" is Hindi and means "wind". Vayu was also a primary Hindu Deity, the Lord of the Winds. So, the sages of earth time in the Indus region, again the region of *Inanna* or *Isis* created exercises to give you one or more of the winds you need to keep your body in tiptop breath. Full of air in motion.

The practice of Yoga is a combination of practices for different purposes. One, you have the postures which are called Asana. Two, you have the breath control which is called *Pranayama*. Then three we have the *Shat Kriyas* which are used to cleanse as well as purify the physical body.

Breath is so important. And I believe the practice of breath exercises can delay or prevent the invasion of disease be it bacteria or virus into your bodies. Can also stop a virus attached to your organs from killing you looking for glucose. Breath gets the blood moving on its run to feed your cells the glucose with its oxygen.

I will now explain to you the five breathing exercises goals. This is a dedicated proactive practice that takes time to learn and perfect. I am only introducing this here and now so you become aware it exists and when you are ready if ever you can use them to make you healthier and wiser.

First up is *Prana Vayu*. This is breath for energy to receive inside your body. To make your body work.

Second is *Alana Aayu*. This is energy that expels outward. This energy, so you are aware, causes sweating and eliminates digestive waste including poisons.

Third is *Samina Vayu*. This is to balance the air and cause the fire of energy to ignite inside our system of circulation.

Fourth is *Udana Vayu*. These exercises are to help or cause your air to move upward in an attempt to help give you clarity of the mind as well as acute sensory functions.

Fifth is *Vyana Vayu*. This practice is to help induce the movement of the air to each body part we have.

When you see the picture presented by these practices you will learn why we must move around. The movement with breath gets the blood flowing. We feed our system. Plants stay still until a wind gets them to move. We have the wind in our body when we learn how to make breath the wind of health and enlightenment.

Now I feel I have stated my case let me recap. We are responsible for our lives as well as responsible to help each other as we are all one common tribe of consciousness invading earth from the beyond and in this dimension we broke into separate individual parts. In this shattered form we have EGO's where we edged GOD out to be able to try and play physical life as someone's boss.

To live here on earth as the tribe of human consciousness we must share information. We must end the game of private ownership of wisdom as well as current knowledge of how and why we can survive living amongst each other as a community of mankind on this planet.

We came as one consciousness and tried to make this dimension the heaven we all dream about and believe in. But now after living here we believe others who say "follow my lead and next time you can go to heaven and sit with God. But you must obey and do as I the self -proclaimed representative of god tells you".

We left God to experience life in physical form as I said. If we try and learn to love each other and work together with transparency, the key I believe, is that we can make this planet our Heaven. Heaven will again appear by following the rules of Earth in how our bodies are created and what we must do to keep our bodies alive on Earth.

Our collective consciousness before we separated into individual parts called beings saw Earth from the beyond. We came to Earth and joined a physical form to experience the physical sensations of having life in a physical body. These physical with spiritual sensations must be geared to have our earth amusement park joys of living and learning to live love in the way Father God wishes and Mother Earth intended us to play. We need to remember that Mother Earth owns this amusement park. We do not.

With love and gratitude, I say Sat Nam.

Poem 2

Deeply inhale
And hold it inside
Let the breath rise up
To unveil your third eye

Let the air out
With a fiery breath
Cleansing your body
Till no illness is left

Put your hands up
To your sacred heart
Take a deep breath
So meditation can start

Open your eyes
And gaze down at your nose
Chanting *"Wahe Guru"*
As you're holding the pose

Open your chakras
To let the light in
With love as your guide
To your power within

Kundalini practice
pathway to your health
There's no greater gift
It's spiritual true wealth

Your inner peace
Will keep your life whole
Don't let a virus
Take over your soul

- Debbie Veltri

Appendix A:

First set of poses

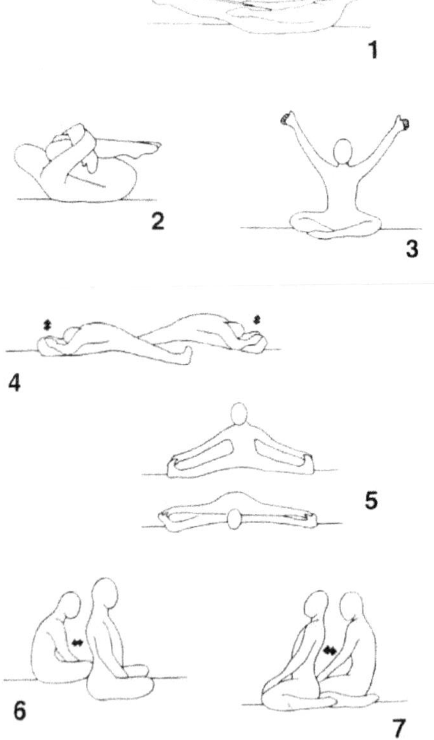

AWAKENING YOURSELF TO YOUR TEN BODIES

1. Stretch Pose – Lie on your back with your arms at your sides. Raise the head and the legs six inches, and the hands six inches with the palms facing each other slightly over the hips to build energy across the navel point. Point the toes, keep your eyes focused on the tips of the toes and do Breath of Fire. 1–3 minutes.

2. Bring the knees to the chest, with the arms wrapped around the knees. Tuck the nose between the knees, and begin Breath of Fire. 1–3 minutes.

3. Sit in Celibate Pose or Easy Pose. Raise the arms to a 60 degree angle, with the fingers tucked into the mounds of the hands. Keep the thumbs pointing up. Eyes closed, concentrate at the third eye point and do Breath of Fire. 1–3 minutes.

4. Sit with the legs stretched wide apart. Arms overhead, inhale, then exhale, stretch down and grab the toes of the left foot. Inhale and come up, and then exhale and stretch down over the right leg and grab the toes. Continue 1–3 minutes.

5. Continue to sit with the legs stretched wide apart. Hold onto the toes, inhale and stretch down bringing the forehead to the floor, then exhale and come sitting up. 1–3 minutes.

6. Camel Ride – Sit in Easy Pose. Grab the shins in front with both hands. Inhale. Flex the spine forward and rock forward on buttocks. Then exhale, flex the spine backwards and roll back on buttocks. Keep the head level and arms fairly straight and relaxed. 1–3 minutes.

7. Sit on the heels. Place the hands flat on the thighs. Flex the spine forward on the inhale, backward on the exhale. Focus at the third eye point. 1–3 minutes.

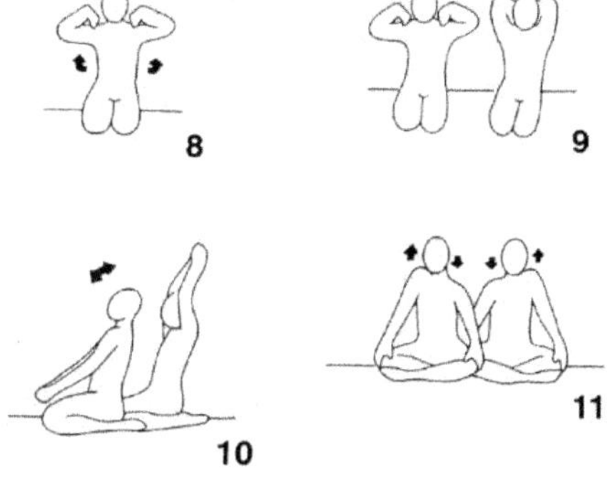

8. Still on the heels, grasp the shoulders with the fingers in front, thumbs in back. Inhale and twist to the left, exhale and twist to the right. Keep the arms parallel to the floor. 1–3 minutes.

9. Grasp the shoulders as in the previous exercise. Inhale and raise the elbows up so that the backs of the wrists touch behind the neck. Exhale and lower the elbows to the original position. 1–3 minutes.

10. Interlace the fingers in Venus lock. Inhale and stretch the arms up over the head, then exhale and bring the hands back to the lap. 1–3 minutes.

11. Sit in Easy Pose with the hands resting on the knees. Inhale and shrug the left shoulder up, then exhale and raise the right shoulder up as you lower the left shoulder. Continue for 1 minute. Then, reverse the breath so that you inhale as you shrug the right shoulder up, exhale as you shrug the left shoulder and lower the right shoulder. Continue for 1 minute.

12. Inhale and shrug both shoulders up, exhale down. 1 minute

13. Remain sitting in Easy Pose hands on the knees. Inhale, and twist your head to the left, and exhale and twist it to the right, like shaking your head "no". Continue for 1 minute. Then reverse your breath, so that you inhale and twist to the right, and exhale and twist to the left. Continue for 1 minute. Inhale deeply, concentrate at the third eye, and slowly exhale.

14. Frog Pose – Squat down so the buttocks are on the heels. The heels are off the ground and touching each other. Put the fingertips on the ground between the knees. Keep the head up. Inhale, straighten legs up, keeping the fingers on the ground. Exhale and come down. The inhale and exhale should be strong. Continue this cycle 54 times.

15. Deeply relax on the back.

Laya Yoga Meditation

Sit in Easy Pose with the hands on the knees in gyan mudra (thumb and index finger together.) Chant "Ek Ong Kar–a, Sat(a) Nam–a, Siri Wha–a Hay Guru." For each underlined word in the mantra, pull up on mul bhand (simultaneously pull up on the rectum and sex organs and pull in on the navel.) This is a 3–1/2 cycle meditation. With the breath, visualize the sound going from the base of the spine to the top of the head in 3 1/2 circles. 11–31 minutes.

Appendix B:

Second set of poses

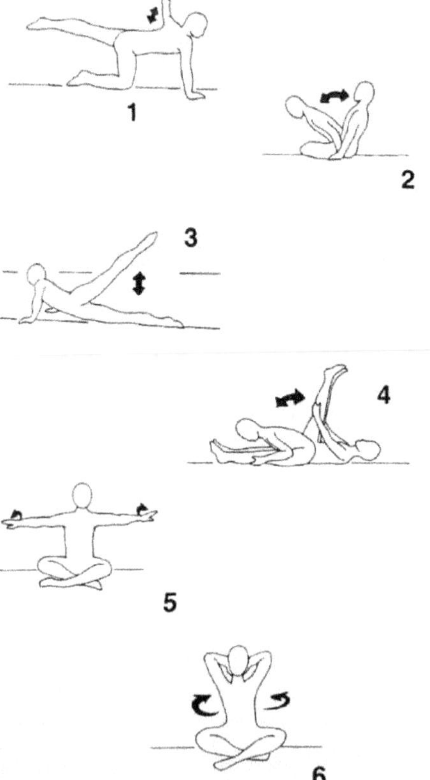

ENERGIZE YOUR SYSTEM

January 5, 1988

1. Kneel on your hands and knees. Raise your left hand up and out to the side at a 60 degree angle. Raise your left leg straight out behind you parallel to the ground. Begin moving the left arm up and down very hard and fast. Your range of movement should be three feet. Your breath will become a powerful navel breath automatically. 2 1/2 minutes.

   This movement energizes the heart and stomach, gives power to the immune system, and stimulates the thyroid and parathyroid. Change sides, lifting the right arm and leg and continue the rapid movement for 1 minute. Change sides again, returning to the original position and continue 30 seconds.

2. Sit in Easy Pose and place your hands palms down on the floor beside your hips. Put your weight on your hands and bend backward and forward as far as you can. (Your body will lift off the floor.) Keep moving without lifting your hands from the floor. 2 1/2 minutes. This movement adjusts the spine.

3. Come into Cobra Pose. Lift your left leg as high as possible, allowing the left hip to lift and twist. Lower the left leg and raise the right leg as high as possible and continue for 3 minutes. Keep your knees straight but allow the hips to lift with the movement. This exercise benefits the liver.

4. Sit down and stretch your legs out forward. With your palms up, grab your legs under the knees and, without bending the knees, roll back onto your back and forward bringing your head to your knees. Continue 2 minutes. This exercise purifies the blood.

5. Sit in Easy Pose with the arms straight out to the sides parallel to the ground. Rotate your arms backward in small circles very rapidly, keeping the elbows straight. 2 1/2 minutes.

6. Still sitting in Easy Pose, lock your hands behind your head and twist left and right from the base of your spine. 1 minute.

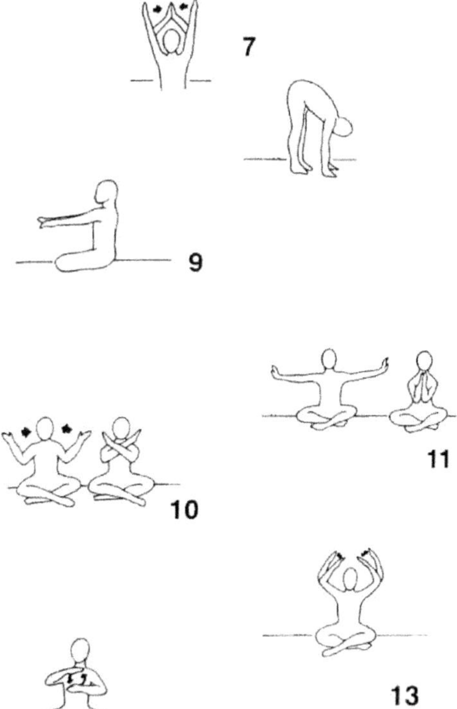

7. Stand up. Place your hands straight over your head and clap, then bend down quickly, keeping the knees straight, and beat the ground with your hands. Continue this movement 108 times.

8. Lie down in Corpse Pose, cover up and relax for 22 minutes. In the class, Yogi Bhajan played the gong and a variety of meditation songs.

9. Stretch the spine and roll the hands and feet. Then sit in Easy Pose and stretch both arms forward, parallel to the ground, with the left palm facing down and the right palm facing upward. Close your eyes and meditate for 3 1/2 minutes.

10. Begin criss-crossing your hands rapidly in front of your body. It's like clapping without touching, the hands pass by each other. 1 1/2 minutes.

11. Stretch your arms out to the sides, parallel to the ground, bend wrists so palms are facing outward, fingertips pointing toward the ceiling. Bring hands to the center of your chest and clap and return to the stretched position. Move quickly. 15 seconds.

12. Begin revolving the hands around each other in front of your chest, moving fast enough to create a breeze which you can feel on your face. 1 minute.

13. Raise your hands over your head and bend the elbows. Begin patting the air above your head as if you were blessing yourself. 1 minute. Inhale and tense the posture, hold the breath for 20 seconds. Exhale, inhale, hold the breath, tense the posture for 20 seconds. Exhale, inhale, tense the posture and hold the breath 15 seconds. Exhale and relax.

9 781649 706065